A pound of prevention ...

The best time to work on managing temper tantrums is when nothing special is happening: You're feeling calm, your child is relaxed, and neither one of you is overtired or on edge. The reason for this is twofold:

1. Kids learn better when they aren't feeling out of control or defensive. Trying to teach a child a better way to behave when he's in the midst of a blowout is like expecting him to understand a movie that's been dubbed in a foreign language: He can see your lips move, but he can't comprehend a word you're saying. Most children are too overwhelmed during a tantrum to even think, never mind listen. Think of how you feel when someone accuses you of doing something wrong. Is your first impulse a desire to deny the wrongdoing or to place the blame elsewhere? It is for many children, and since kids aren't as skilled at controlling their impulses as adults are, they often do just that. . . .

2. Prevention is still the best medicine. Every time you help your child avoid a temper tantrum or master her emotions, you show her that you're on her side—that you want her to feel in control and confident. At the same time, you encourage her to believe that she can control her actions and emotions. . . .

Also from the editors of *Child* magazine

Goodbyes: How to Say "See You Later" to Your
 Little Alligator
Sleep: How to Teach Your Child to Sleep Like a Baby

Published by POCKET BOOKS

From the Editors of **child** Magazine

TANTRUMS

secrets to calming the storm

Ann E. La Forge

A New Century Communications Book

POCKET BOOKS

New York   London   Toronto   Sydney   Tokyo   Singapore

The author of this book is not a physician and the ideas, procedures, and suggestions in this book are not intended as a substitute for the medical advice of a trained health professional. All matters regarding your child's health require medical supervision. Consult your child's physician before adopting the suggestions in this book, as well as about any condition that may require diagnosis or medical attention. The author and publisher disclaim any liability arising directly or indirectly from the use of the book.

An *Original* Publication of POCKET BOOKS

POCKET BOOKS, a division of Simon & Schuster Inc.
1230 Avenue of the Americas, New York, NY 10020

ISBN: 0-671-88039-X

First Pocket Books printing July 1996

10 9 8 7 6 5 4 3 2 1

POCKET and colophon are registered trademarks of Simon & Schuster Inc.

Cover photo by Tosca Radigonda Felicello

Printed in the U.S.A.

962811

To my parents, with gratitude and love

Acknowledgments

This book would not have been possible without the generosity of many people. I'd particularly like to thank the following child-care professionals, who donated their time and expertise during lengthy telephone interviews:

Lawrence Balter, Ph.D., child psychologist and professor of applied psychology at New York University in New York City, and author of *Not in Front of the Children . . . How to Talk to Your Child About Tough Family Matters* and *Who's in Control? Dr. Balter's Guide to Discipline Without Combat*

Karen Buchanan, parent educator for Project Enlightenment, an early intervention program of the Wake County Public School System, based in Raleigh, North Carolina

Stella Chess, M.D., professor of child psychiatry at New York University Medical Center, in New York

City, and author of *Know Your Child: An Authoritative Guide for Today's Parents* and *Temperament in Clinical Practice*

George J. Cohen, M.D., medical director of the general pediatric ambulatory center at Children's National Medical Center in Washington, D.C., and a professor of pediatrics at George Washington University School of Medicine, also in Washington, D.C.

Susan Crockenberg, Ph.D., professor of psychology at the University of Vermont in Burlington

Richard Ferber, M.D., director of the Center for Pediatric Sleep Disorders at Children's Hospital in Boston, assistant professor of neurology at Harvard Medical School, and author of *Solve Your Child's Sleep Problems*

Stephen W. Garber, Ph.D., clinical behavioral psychologist and director of the Behavioral Institute of Atlanta and coauthor (with Marianne Daniels Garber, Ph.D., and Robyn Freedman Spizman) of *Good Behavior* and *Monsters Under the Bed and Other Childhood Fears*

Barbara J. Howard, M.D., assistant clinical professor of pediatrics at Duke University Medical Center, in Durham, North Carolina, and advisor for Learning Through Entertainment, which produces the Duke Family Series of educational videotapes for children and parents

Karen L. Johnson, M.S.Ed., CCC-SLD, certified speech-language pathologist with the South Windsor Public School System in Connecticut

Jerome Kagan, Ph.D., professor of psychology at Harvard University, in Cambridge, Massachusetts

Kathy A. Merritt, M.D., assistant professor in the

division of general pediatrics at Duke University Medical Center, in Durham, North Carolina, and a private practitioner with Chapel Hill Pediatrics, P.A., Chapel Hill, North Carolina

Mary Rothbart, Ph.D., professor of psychology at the University of Oregon, in Eugene, and coauthor (with Holly Ruf) of *Attention in Early Development: Themes and Variations*

Nancy Samalin, founder of Parent Guidance workshops in New York City and coauthor (with Catharine Whitney) of *Love and Anger: The Parental Dilemma*

Marilyn Segal, Ph.D., developmental psychologist and dean of the Family and School Center at Nova Southeastern University in Fort Lauderdale, Florida

Betty Smith Franklin, Ph.D., associate professor of psychology at Goucher College in Towson, Maryland

Stanley Turecki, M.D., child and family psychiatrist, director of the Difficult Child Center in New York City, and coauthor (with Leslie Tonner) of *The Difficult Child* and (with Sarah Wernick) of *The Emotional Problems of Normal Children*

Peter Williamson, Ph.D., child psychologist at the Dean Medical Center in Madison, Wisconsin, and author of *Good Kids, Bad Behavior*

James Windell, M.A., clinical psychologist with the Oakland County Juvenile Court Psychological Clinic in Oakland County, Michigan, and author of *Discipline: A Sourcebook of 50 Failsafe Techniques for Parents* and *8 Weeks to a Well-Behaved Child*

Thanks also to:

The American Academy of Pediatrics, for providing background materials and referring me to experts.

Rosalyn Alexander, Darcy Berger, Tekla Jachimiak, and Nancy Sparrow of the Duke School for Children in Durham, North Carolina, for broadening my perspective and understanding of young children during informal conversations and parent-training seminars.

Frank Dobisky and Associates, Keene, New Hampshire, for putting me in touch with child-care experts at universities around the country.

I am also indebted to the many wise parents who were willing not only to admit that their kids threw temper tantrums, but to fill out a long questionnaire on the subject, and share their experiences during follow-up interviews:

Margot Adler, Henry Cunningham, Carolyn Davenport, Elizabeth Dunn, Trudy Eaton, Holly Hughes, Samantha Hughes, Donna Kerbel, Suzanne Koller, Janice O'Brien, Kelly Smith, Carol Spelman, Patricia Sutter, Kathy Turlington, Wendy White-Hensen, and many other parents who asked to remain anonymous.

I am also grateful to Peggy Schmidt of New Century Communications, the editors of *Child* magazine, and Claire Zion of Pocket Books for their support and guidance.

Last but not least, I thank my husband and children for their invaluable input, unflagging patience, and incomparable love.

Contents

LETTER FROM THE EDITOR   xiii

INTRODUCTION
*The Birthday Boy Throws a
Tantrum*   xv

ONE
The Tantrum Years   1

TWO
The Role of Temperament   28

THREE
*Parents, Pitfalls, and Problem
Solving*   57

FOUR
A Pound of Prevention   84

FIVE

A Ton of Cure   128

SIX

Happy Endings   160

RESOURCES   177

Letter from the Editor

Dear Reader:

Expectant parents are quick to fill their shelves with books to prepare them for what's to come. But once the baby arrives, moms and dads are more likely to turn to information that's accessible, to the point, and a quick read. We created the *Child* Magazine Series for Parents for just that reason.

What makes the *Child* Magazine Series for Parents unique is that each book is intended to help parents of young children—babies, toddlers, preschoolers, and early school-age children—deal with a specific problem—quickly. The books are written by accomplished journalists who have picked the brains of leading child psychologists, researchers, and child-care experts and organized their collective wisdom. The benefit to you is that you will be presented with a number of strategies for understanding and coping with your child's behavior. You can select the one that best suits your parenting style, or try more than one if the first one you choose doesn't achieve the change you're looking for.

If you're a busy parent who needs help *now* to solve the problem featured in this book, I hope you will pick it up and start reading it tonight. I'm sure that the small investment of your time will provide a quick return as you implement the solutions we present. Throughout the book, you will find age "flags" that will help you easily find the sections that relate most directly to your situation. And if you find this advice helpful, try another book in this series; each one is written in the same friendly, informative style as *Child* magazine articles.

We'd love to hear from you after you have read the book. Let us know what worked for you, and whether you have any additional ideas that we might include in future editions of this book. Write to us at: *Child, Child* Magazine Series for Parents, 110 Fifth Avenue, New York, NY 10003. Or e-mail us at: Childmag@aol.com.

Pamela Abrams
Editor-in-Chief

Introduction

The Birthday Boy Throws a Tantrum

It was supposed to be a happy day. My son Gus was turning 4, and I had planned a birthday party crammed with things I knew he'd enjoy: pirate bandannas, face painting, and a pirate piñata, as well as balloons and bubble wands to go around, apple juice, cupcakes, and ice cream; plus favors and treats for his friends to take home. I thought I had thought of everything—and was fully expecting my grateful son to take as much pleasure in the party as I had taken in planning it.

I must have been dreaming. No sooner did the first guest arrive than Gus began begging to open his presents. He couldn't have cared less if we were on a deserted island with nothing to eat but bananas and coconut milk: he wanted those toys, and he wanted them *now!* The more I tried to distract him, the angrier he got, until finally, he snapped. He flung himself across the decorated picnic table and, in his most pitiful voice, began wailing to get his way.

It wasn't his first temper tantrum—nor, unfortunately, his last—but it was, for me, one of his most embarrassing. The kids stopped playing, the parents stopped talking, and all eyes turned to Gus; then they turned to me. I wanted to disappear. Not only was I embarrassed by my son's behavior, I felt angry at him for spoiling the party. I felt guilty for not having prevented the tantrum; and I felt sad that he was feeling so distressed. But I had to act, so I did exactly what you're never supposed to do: I gave in (after all, he was the birthday boy) and let him open his presents first.

The good news is that the party was a breeze after that, and everyone had a wonderful time. The bad news: I hadn't gotten any closer to helping my son control his temper—and he wasn't getting any younger. I was certain that somehow it was all my fault. My friends' kids never threw tantrums (at least not when I was around, and certainly not at their own birthday parties). Where had I gone wrong? I wondered. Was I a terrible parent? Was my son abnormal? Did other parents know something I didn't know about child rearing? Would the tantrums ever end?

If you have a child who throws frequent or intense temper tantrums, you probably know exactly what I was going through. And you've probably asked yourself the same types of questions over and over again.

I want you to know that you're not alone. All parents—no matter how perfect their children seem—must face and survive the tantrum years (which last from about 15 months old to age 5 or 6). "This is a period of intense emotional, physical, and cognitive growth for children," explains Lawrence Balter, Ph.D., a child psychologist based in New York City and author of *Who's in Control? Dr. Balter's Guide to Discipline Without Combat.* "Tantrums are a natural by-product." In fact, some experts say they worry more about the child who never throws tantrums than the ones who do.

Why? Because tantrums enable young kids to do some very healthy things, such as assert their independence, express their individuality, voice their opinion, vent their anger and frustration, blow off steam, and let adults know when they're overstimulated, overwhelmed, overly tired, or sick. Granted, kicking, screaming, and flailing about aren't the prettiest forms of communication, but for children who haven't acquired the words to express their emotions or mastered the art of self-control, they get the job done.

Tantrums also help children test their boundaries—does my mommy or daddy really mean no? what will happen if I keep on crying and complaining? can I get away with breaking this?—which, in turn, helps them to learn.

"Misbehavior is one of the healthiest activities of childhood," says Peter Williamson, Ph.D., a child psychologist based in Madison, Wisconsin, and author of *Good Kids, Bad Behavior.* "It enables kids to learn how to regulate themselves, and sharpens their ability to predict how others will respond to them. The better they get at predicting, the more they can set limits on their own behavior and improve their self-control."

That's not to say tantrums should be encouraged or praised, however. If a child's experiments with tantrums reveal that they work—they get her what she wants, when she wants it—she can quickly learn to use them to manipulate as well as communicate. Unfortunately, this is what gives tantrums such a bad rap—and why parents tend to fear them or feel ashamed when they happen.

No one wants to be responsible for raising a spoiled brat, so instead of seeing tantrum behavior for what it is—a normal part of development—many adults view it as a threat. We ascribe adult motives to the behavior ("she's just doing this to annoy me"; "he's looking for attention"; "she never listens to anything I say") and react with anger, frustration, and resentment. Or we feel so discomfited by the intensity of the child's rage (thinking "I wouldn't act like that unless I was really, really upset") that we back down on perfectly reasonable requests and limits.

When tantrums happen in public, we feel embarrassed and ashamed—of both our kids and ourselves. We remember all the times (before we had children) when we saw distraught parents yelling at overwrought kids in department stores and thought, "What a terrible parent—I'd never do that to my kid"—and assume everyone else is thinking the same about us. Then we feel guilty, and fear everyone else is right. ("It is all my fault. I made him throw the tantrum, or I should have handled it better.")

When tantrums don't happen in public or around other caregivers—only at home, and only around us—we really feel like failures. We can't help wondering things like, "Why is she doing this to me? What did I ever do to make her hate me so much?"

The truth is, parents do not cause temper tantrums, and if you have a tantrum-prone child, it's not your fault. Your child's inborn temperament and stage of development—both of which you have little control over—play key roles in determining the frequency and intensity of her outbursts.

But you can—and should—make a difference in how your child manages his temper. Even though tantrums are a normal part of development, they can be scary for kids. They feel like a huge internal explosion that the child can neither control nor comprehend. The burst of rage and other violent feelings take him over, body and soul. Whether he runs around the room screaming, flings himself onto the floor to kick and cry, flails about and breaks everything in his path, or holds his breath until he faints, the experience is not pleasant. And although we adults know that all tantrums eventually end, a child who is in the midst of one doesn't necessarily understand that, and may fear his intense feelings will continue forever.

Also, if you allow tantrums free reign, or react to them with too much force or harsh punishment, you simply model and encourage the aggressive behavior you're trying to stop. Plus, you lose out on some valuable opportunities to teach your child how to cope with normal emotions—like anger, jealousy, frustration, and fear—and how to behave in a way that won't harm or frighten him or others.

I'm not going to mislead you and say there's a sure cure for all temper tantrums. I know from my own experience with two wonderful—but temperamental—sons that there's no quick fix. As with any parenting problem, it takes a continuous stream of time and patience to teach a child self-control. But you *can* learn better ways to handle your child's tantrums and to manage yourself when they happen. This, in turn, will reduce the quantity, intensity, and long-term impact of tantrums in your household.

The key comes in understanding why your child behaves as she does, and why you react as you do. Once you put these into perspective, you can let go of your worries and guilt, and concentrate on ways to teach positive alternatives to losing control.

In this book, you'll find the information and tools you need to begin. Chapter One features an overview of what to expect tantrum-wise at different ages. Understanding that certain types of misbehavior are both normal and healthy during a child's earliest years of life is essential. It will help you step back from tantrums and see them from your child's standpoint, rather than from your own. Chapter Two reviews some important thinking on temperament, and the role it plays in tantrums. Chapter Three looks at the parent's contribution—both positive and negative—to the tantrum process. And Chapters Four and Five offer step-by-step strategies on how to prevent tantrums, how to react when they're in progress, and how to teach a lesson once they're over.

Finally, in Chapter Six—my favorite—you'll find out what other parents have experienced and what they've learned from dealing with kids who throw tantrums. These real-life examples are both reassuring and instructive.

The research and advice offered in this book come from an intensive review of existing literature on temper tantrums, plus in-depth interviews with experts—including child psychologists, pediatricians, daycare and preschool teachers, and researchers. In addition, there are stories and insights from parents who have gone through exactly what you're going through and emerged with relatively well-behaved kids. (For a complete list of contributors, please see Acknowledgments on page vii.) I know that I have benefited from all their advice and experiences—and I hope you will, too.

Remember, parenting may be one of the most difficult and thankless jobs on this planet, but it also happens to be the most important. And the fact that you are reading this book means that your child already has the one thing she needs most: a parent who cares.

TANTRUMS

❀ ONE

The Tantrum Years

"I'll never forget my daughter Whitney's first temper tantrum," says Samantha Hughes, director of an in-home daycare. "She was not quite 2 years old, and we were driving from North Carolina to Boston with Nick and Laura (two of the children I was caring for at the time), and their parents, Bob and Ruthanne. We stopped at a Roy Rogers to get some lunch, and at the entrance there were some flashy video games that caught Whitney's eye.

"I tried to guide her past the games to the food counter, but she wanted to stay, so she started hooting and hollering, stamping her feet, and demanding that I let her play the games. When I finally got her into the booth beside me, she wriggled out of the seat, snuck under the table, and shot straight for those video games. She was like a maniac.

"I was shocked—she had never acted that way before—and embarrassed. Here I was, unable to control

1

my own daughter, while the people I babysat for were looking on. Plus, she was being so loud that her tantrum was ruining other diners' meals. Nothing I did could calm her down, so I finally gave in and let Bob take her over to the games while the rest of us ate. That ended the tantrum, but we hadn't been on the road for more than 3 minutes when Whitney started complaining she was hungry."

Sound familiar? Like Samantha, many parents are caught totally off guard by that first temper tantrum and don't quite know how to react. One minute they have a compliant infant, the next minute, a defiant toddler—and they haven't the faintest idea why. As one parent put it: "My son changed so suddenly that I felt like someone must have switched kids on me in the middle of the night."

Other parents barely even notice that first tantrum because their child has been so vocal and expressive since birth. "I don't have a clear memory of Zack's first tantrum," says Carolyn Davenport, a mother of two. "They just sort of crept up on me. I know they started early, though, because I have a photograph of me holding Zack in a swimming pool. He is about 13 months old, and he's arching his back, screaming about something. At that point, I didn't call such behavior a tantrum—I called it being a baby. By the time he was 18 months old, however, I had no doubt that Zack was throwing tantrums."

Typical Tantrum Behaviors

Tantrums and temper outbursts take many different forms. Here are some of the most common—and normal—behaviors you may witness.

Under age 3:

- Crying
- Biting
- Hitting
- Kicking
- Screaming
- Screeching
- Arching the back
- Throwing self on floor
- Pounding or flailing arms
- Breath-holding
- Head-banging
- Throwing things

Ages 3 to 4—any of the above, plus:

- Stomping
- Yelling
- Whining
- Criticizing
- Shaking clenched fists
- Slamming doors
- Accidentally breaking things

Age 5 and up—any of the above, plus:

- Swearing
- Self-criticism
- Striking out at a sibling or friend
- Deliberately breaking things
- Threatening

Ten Top Tantrum Triggers

1. Frustration
2. Fatigue
3. Hunger
4. Illness

5. Anger
6. Jealousy
7. Changes in routine
8. Stress at home (from divorce, moving, death, chronic illness, financial problems, and so on)
9. Stress at school (social or academic)
10. Insecurity (about self or abilities)

Whether you notice it or not, most kids, like Whitney and Zack, throw their first temper tantrum sometime between the ages of 1 or 2. Typically, the child wants something very, very badly—a certain object or toy, a chance to run free in the supermarket, a special food that's out of reach—but he can't have it or can't reach it, so he explodes in frustration and rage. Depending on his personal style, he may cry, scream, kick, arch his back, throw himself on the floor, pound the table, bite you, bang his head against a wall, or hold his breath until he turns blue. It's never a pretty sight, but that first temper tantrum is an important milestone: It indicates that your child is developing normally.

Understanding this is a crucial first step in helping your child tame her temper. Contrary to popular myth, tantrums are not a sign that your child is "bad" or "spoiled," and they can't be remedied with harsh punishment. They are a natural part of a vital developmental process, and should be treated with understanding and love.

To help you put your child's temper outbursts into perspective, here is an overview of tantrum behavior in normal children, from birth to age six.

EARLY TANTRUMS

AGE FLAG: BIRTH TO 2 YEARS

Most newborns are pretty much content to let their parents run the show. They'll go along with whatever you decide in terms of where they sleep, who gets to hold them, what they eat, when they go outside for a walk, and what they wear—but only for a while. Sometime after their 6-month birthday, they inevitably decide they want considerably more say. They don't exactly have tantrums quite yet, but if you take a toy away in the middle of play, they'll cry to get it back; if they don't like the way their lunch looks, they'll toss it in your face; and if you put them in the playpen when they want to be on the floor, they'll pitch a fit until someone picks them up.

These are early signs that your child is discovering she's a separate being, with opinions and desires all her own. They signal a critical new objective for her, one that will play a central role throughout her early childhood: independence.

As a baby begins to crawl and then walk, this objective grows into something of an obsession. Suddenly, the child can move across a room and reach for whatever he wants without anyone else's help. This new freedom is incredibly exciting—and terrifying. On the one hand, the child is feeling: "free at last—I'm free at last"; on the other: "help. Don't leave me. This is too scary." Both emotions are enormously powerful, and kids this age spend much of their time shifting back and forth, from one to another, all day long. By the time a baby is 15 or 16 months old, every little decision—should I stay or should I go? should I touch that or leave it alone? should I roll the ball or throw it?—becomes part of that inner struggle between autonomy and dependence.

This is the point at which tantrums usually begin. For parents, it's a time of confusion. Your baby may cry to be picked up, for instance, but as soon as you pick her up, she'll cry to be put down; as soon as you put her down, she'll cry to be picked up again. Or she'll point excitedly at something she wants, and if you can't figure out what it is fast enough, she'll dissolve into tears.

Anything from a broken cookie to a dropped doll can trigger a full-blown tantrum, and outbursts may be so intense that they leave your child exhausted and you dazed. Half the time, you don't even know what started a tantrum or what your child really wants.

In many cases, your child doesn't know, either. All he knows is that he doesn't want you to control his life anymore, yet he wants to remain your pampered baby; he's determined to do his own thing, but he doesn't want to make you angry; he craves adventure and wants to take risks, but he's afraid of what might happen if he doesn't play it safe.

Most children can't handle the stress of all this inner turmoil for very long. Their coping mechanisms are rudimentary, at best, and their communication skills are primitive. Little by little, their fears, frustrations, and disappointments accumulate, until they're so emotionally charged, they explode.

"When my 15-month-old is in the midst of a full-blown tantrum, it seems like he's lost not only his self-control, but his self," says Henry Cunningham, a father of two boys. "Rather than being a person with emotions of varying intensities, he becomes a site in which runaway emotions—rage, helplessness, grief—take over and get all jumbled up; he's like an incoherent mass of impulses."

Henry, like many other parents, finds it difficult to watch these out-of-control tantrums. They conjure up too many uncomfortable feelings, such as guilt (that somehow you caused the tantrum), anger (that the child is being so defiant when you've tried so hard to please her), resentment (that she's ruining everyone else's good time), fear (that she might hurt herself or grow up to be a maniac), and helplessness (because nothing you do seems to calm her down).

"When my oldest son, Hugh, used to have tantrums, we'd call them 'meltdowns,' because that's what would happen," says Holly Hughes, a mother of three. "All of his systems would collapse at once, and he'd just spin out of control. This usually made me melt down, too. I'd get completely tense, panicky, and anxious. I'd even break into a sweat. And I'd feel furious at everyone else—at my husband for not being home, at my babysitter for leaving early, at the telemarketers for phoning during dinnertime—I'd blame anyone I could for making it worse."

Aside from arousing uncomfortable emotions and irrational thoughts, early tantrums can make us seriously doubt our parenting skills—especially if we're dealing with a first child.

"Zack's tantrums used to make me feel so helpless and guilty," says Carolyn Davenport. "He was my first child, so I thought I had done something basically wrong to cause them. I thought maybe I was working and traveling too much, and not spending enough one-on-one time with him. Or maybe I was being too strict—or too permissive. I was constantly second-guessing myself, and questioning my ability to be a good parent."

Fortunately, these kinds of fears are usually unfounded. "Early tantrums are normal, healthy, and, to a great extent, unavoidable," explains George J. Cohen, M.D., medical director of the general pediatric ambulatory center at Children's National Medical Center in Washington, D.C. They do not indicate that you are a bad parent, or that you have an abnormal or unusually bad child. They do not prove your child is out to get you. And most of all, they do not foretell a future filled with violence and aggression for your kid. (Many hot-tempered toddlers grow up to be calm, well-adjusted adults, while some easy-going 2-year-olds wait until their teens to act out and rebel.)

Even if your child throws more than her share of tantrums—outdoing your friends', neighbors', and even a sibling's kids—you needn't be too concerned. While all children pass through this stage of negativity, the range of normal behavior is quite wide, and is easily influenced by factors like environment, stress level, and temperament.

In general, kids who were calm, easy-to-please babies tend to attempt only a few minor tantrums in this stage; those who were unpredictable, reacted strongly to change, resisted anything new, or were difficult to calm and satisfy, will likely erupt more often and more intensely. (Chapter Two explores the role of temperament in great detail.)

If your child is of the hot-tempered variety, your job as a parent may be more challenging, but your kid has as good a chance of learning to behave as anyone else. Tantrum-prone children aren't—as many adults believe—"rotten" or "spoiled." In fact, it's far more likely they are intelligent, creative, artistic, or sensitive. The worst you can say is that they're tiny people with strong ideas about what they want and a capacity for great disappointment when they're thwarted, frustrated, or refused.

"In American culture, there's this mythical notion that 'normal' means even-tempered," adds Stephen W. Garber, Ph.D., clinical behavioral psychologist and director of the Behavioral Institute of Atlanta, in Georgia. "We think that when a child is highly sensitive, strong-willed, or stubborn, it's a bad thing. But ironically, the qualities that cause problems in childhood often end up being the strengths that help people lead and succeed as adults."

Whether your baby has many tantrums or just a few, then, it's important to remember that the only thing these early outbursts really indicate is that she's begun the process of growing up, communicating how she feels, and controlling her emotions. You help her most when you view them with patience, sympathy, and support.

TODDLER TANTRUMS

AGE FLAG: 2 TO 3 YEARS

As your child matures, tantrums are likely to get worse before they get better. Aside from being creative, charming, and adorable, 2-year-olds are known for being active, stubborn, noisy, impulsive, easily distracted, and uncooperative. Whether it's bathtime, bedtime, dinnertime, or playtime, they love to say *"no!"*—even when they really mean yes—and when things don't go the way they want or plan, they often feel outraged. Welcome to the "terrible twos."

Not surprisingly, this is a peak period for temper tantrums. The struggle between dependence and independence is in full swing by now, but coping and communication skills remain way under par. Until these lines connect, trouble looms.

Almost anything can trigger a tantrum in a 2-year-old, and often there is no rational cause. One parent remembers his child throwing a tantrum because he gave her an ice cream cone she had begged for; another recalls an outburst over putting on shoes before playing outdoors. In most cases, however, toddler tantrums occur because the child is feeling overwhelmed by his emotions, environment, or activities, and needs a way to blow off steam.

Common Causes of Frustration in Kids Aged 1 to 5 Years Old

* Can't verbalize feelings or desires
* Can't coordinate body and mind (as when drawing a picture or trying to throw a ball or ride a bike)
* Can't get others to do what he wants
* Toys are too complicated
* Can't sit still for long periods (in a car, at a store, during a visit to Grandma's, and so forth)
* Isn't allowed to touch anything in a store or other place filled with new and interesting things
* Isn't allowed to try to do something all by himself

* Feels rushed or isn't allowed to dawdle, explore, or play enough
* Has too many planned activities in her day
* Can't understand an adult's instructions or requests
* Is uncertain of an adult's expectations
* Has to stop playing to eat or go to bed

It's incredibly easy to push a kid this young too far—and not even realize it, until it's too late. One reason is that many of the things toddlers consider quite exciting, we adults consider boring or mundane. We assume that a trip to the post office or bank, for example, is no big deal. But when you're only 2 years old, everything's a big deal—even something as ordinary as riding in the car or standing in a line.

Unfortunately, the average toddler's threshold for new stimulation is usually much lower than her appetite, and sensory overload can occur quickly, with little warning. This is especially likely if your child is already weakened by hunger, fatigue, illness, or stress (from moving, meeting a new sibling, getting a new caregiver, having a parent who is ill or absent, watching parents go through a divorce, and so on). All four of the above, in fact, are major tantrum triggers for kids of any age. (Come to think of it, how many grown-ups do you know can maintain perfect control when they're hungry, tired, worried, or sick?)

It's not just "bad" stress that turns sweet, smiling toddlers into tearful, tyrannical tots, either: happy occasions—such as birthday parties, family reunions, and holiday celebrations—can also push 2-year-olds quickly over the edge. As one mother of a toddler confesses: "I used to love Christmas—until I had a kid. Now I dread it. My daughter gets so overexcited by all of our festivities, decorations, and guests that she ends up throwing nonstop tantrums. They're as common as candy canes in our house, from the time the tree goes up until the day we take it down."

Again, most toddlers simply can't handle too much newness or change. In fact, many of them feel upset every single time they have to make a transition (when moving from one activity to another, such as going to the park/coming home from the park, getting into the car/getting out of the car, greeting a babysitter/leaving a babysitter, or ending playtime to eat or nap).

Part of the problem is that kids this young don't have a clear sense of time; nor do they think ahead. They live for the moment, and if the moment is good (they figure), why ruin it by doing something else? Another reason, however, is that sudden changes feel threatening to young children—they don't know what's going to happen next, they don't like being bossed around, and they're afraid of losing control.

Tempers also tend to flare when a toddler can't have her own way, can't make herself understood, or can't understand what a grownup expects, says Dr. Cohen. The reason is pure frustration. Unlike adults, 2-year-olds don't have sufficient language skills to voice or discuss strong feelings. Many of them can only talk in two-or three-word telegraphic sentences—saying, for example, "Mommy bye-bye" when they really mean, "Oh please, Mommy, take me to the park before I go crazy from being cooped up inside this house all day!" Also, their pronunciation of words is still so iffy that up to half of what they say may not be understood by listeners who aren't part of their immediate family circle.

The most effective communication tools at their disposal are their body and voice, so just as they'll dance, laugh, and clap their hands when they're happy or excited, they'll scream, hit, and kick if they're furious or frightened. In general, the more intense or sensitive the child, and the more passionate her feelings, the more extreme her (positive and negative) behavior will be.

Whether your toddler throws one tantrum a year or 10 tantrums a day, however, one thing is certain: you and/or your spouse will be targeted as his main audience. Kids who are practically perfect in front of grandparents or babysitters routinely cry and run away from their parents when they come to pick them up, or throw rip-roaring tantrums within minutes of arriving home.

"When my daughter, Jane, started throwing tantrums at around age 2, she jumped into it big time, with an average of 8 to 10 a day," says Sharon Johnson (not her real name). "But when I asked her babysitter how she was handling all those outbursts, she just looked at me with disbelief and said, 'Jane? Throwing tantrums? No way!' I felt like crying. It was proof to me I was doing something wrong."

Carol Spelman recalls a similar feeling: "When my daughter Grace first started throwing tantrums, she tried them at the babysitters', as well as at home. But they soon ended at the babysitters'—and increased at home. So I asked the caregiver what her strategy was. She told me she just said, 'Now Gracie, stop it. I'm not going to talk to you until you finish screaming.'

And Grace would stop screaming. I even had her demonstrate the tone of voice she used, so I could try it at home, but when I did the exact same thing, using the same words and tone of voice, it only made Grace more furious, and worsened her tantrum. I felt so frustrated!

"My daughter is an absolute angel when she's around anybody else," adds Carol, "but around me and my husband, she really cuts loose."

Most kids are like Jane and Grace: they behave far worse around their parents—but not because they're angrier with them or because they hate them. Children simply feel safer saving up their fears and frustrations until they're around someone they're sure won't abandon them. Misbehaving may not be your idea of showing trust and love, but if you read between the lines of your child's outbursts, that's what you'll find.

Even so, toddler tantrums are bound to try your patience. They may even embarrass you, infuriate you, or drive you to distraction, but they shouldn't make you feel like a failure. Like early tantrums, they are as normal and necessary at this age as crawling and babbling are in infancy. They indicate nothing more than that your child is learning and growing.

———————————— ✳ ————————————

Warning Signs That Something's Really Wrong

"Normal" has a broad definition when it comes to early and toddler tantrums. At one end is the child who throws mild tantrums every now and then; at the other end, the kid who has a riotous outburst more than once a day.

Either way, you needn't worry that tantrums signal an underlying emotional disorder, unless they are accompanied by an extreme version of any one of the following behaviors:

1. Your child never throws tantrums. In some (though not all) cases, children who don't throw tantrums are repressing their age-appropriate desire for independence. If your child seems unusually passive or "too good" to be true, talk to your pediatrician or a child psychologist.
2. Other children shun her. While it's normal for 2-year-olds to play independently, if other kids seem to purposely avoid yours, there may be cause for concern.
3. He seems indifferent to new stimulations. Most toddlers have a strong reaction—either positive or negative—to new things in their life. Total indifference may signal withdrawal or depression.
4. Her reactions often seem hysterical, extreme, or inappropriate (e.g., one minute she's throwing a violent tantrum, the next minute she's laughing hysterically, then she's suddenly looking vacant). Normal toddlers can be moody, but their behavior is rarely that extreme.
5. He often acts sad for no apparent reason or seems depressed. These are not normal emotions for children; they should be evaluated by a professional.

Even if they look awful, they don't cause lasting damage. Think about what typically happens when a tantrum is over: does your child sulk for the rest of the afternoon, as an adult might? Does she act as though the entire day is ruined beyond repair? Probably not. Two-year-olds may be honest and direct about their anger, but they rarely hold a grudge, and once a tantrum has run its course, they're usually feeling fresh and lively.

"When Hugh's toddler tantrums were over, even if his cheeks were still red and wet from crying, he'd move on to another activity and act like nothing happened," says Holly Hughes. "That helped me see that there's no reason for me to hang on to the angry feelings a tantrum generates. Once it's over, it's over."

No matter how embarrassing, infuriating, or bewildering a toddler's tantrums are, then, don't try to stop them, or to control one that's already begun. Instead, when they happen, accept them, and let them run their course. Then, when things are calm, find ways to cut down on undue frustration in your child's life, and help her learn the coping and communication skills she lacks. (We explore some specific strategies for this in Chapters Four and Five.)

The more you can focus on managing—rather than punishing—when tantrums occur, the more likely it is that your child will emerge from the terrible twos tantrum-free.

PRESCHOOL TANTRUMS

AGE FLAG: 3 TO 4 YEARS

If you're lucky, your child's tantrums will end right around her third birthday. With their growing verbal skills, greater life experience, and increased physical competency, many preschool kids feel less inclined to act out their emotions and more inclined to speak their minds. But don't be surprised—or alarmed—if your child just begins throwing tantrums in the preschool years or maintains a pattern begun earlier. There is nothing magical about a birthday: it doesn't make a child instantly mature.

Preschool-age kids get overtired, hungry, sick, and bored, just like toddlers. And, like everyone else, they tend to fall back on immature coping mechanisms (such as tantrums) when feeling overwhelmed or under stress—which may be quite frequently.

From an adult's perspective, a child's first years of life look pretty easy. After all, kids don't have any work, family, or financial pressures to drag them down, and there's usually someone around to cook them meals and wash their clothes. From a child's view, however, life isn't all cake and ice cream. It takes a lot of hard work and frustration to learn the basics, such as how to walk, talk, get dressed, feed yourself, use the toilet, and make friends.

The preschool years can be especially challenging. This is when most children take their first real steps outside the safety of their homes. They leave the warm embrace of their mother, father, or favorite babysitter, and head off for the wonderful—sometimes bewildering—world of preschool. There, they have to adjust to a new environment, new routines, and a new teacher all at once, plus learn how to play and socialize with all those other kids.

Their uneven development can also cause stress. Though by now, most kids have the cognitive ability to understand how things work, imitate others, and plan and carry out complex ideas, their verbal and physical abilities often fall short of their desires. A kid who makes up a great story or has an exciting idea may not have the language skills to share it with anyone; he may long to hop on a bike like his older cousin, but lack the proper coordination to balance himself and pedal; or he may want to play with a toy that he clearly understands, but simply can't manipulate.

It's bad enough when an adult prevents a child from doing something he wants to do (like run into the street or open a toy box in the store), but when his own body refuses to cooperate, the frustration can be agonizing.

I remember when my son, Gus, first discovered drawing at around age 3. He'd scribble for a while, then, in frustration, hand the paper to me or my husband and ask us to draw the picture in his mind. We'd patiently listen to his description and attempt to comply, but if we, too, fell short of his vision—making the pirate's sword too small or putting the hook on the wrong hand—he'd fly into a rage. As soon as his own skill in drawing improved, these tantrums completely disappeared.

Kids like Gus are not born knowing how to deal with this kind of frustration. They don't have the words to express it or the perspective to accept it. If you're foolish enough to tell them to wait a few years and try something again when they're older, they'll think you've gone insane. From a preschooler's point of view, it's much easier—and more effective—to throw a tantrum than to ponder something that might happen years down the road; for all the kid knows, she may be little for the rest of her life.

As with toddler tantrums, a preschool tantrum that can be closely linked to hunger, fatigue, illness, or frustration is not a cause for serious concern. However, if tantrums are frequent, you may need to evaluate your child's environment and schedule to see what else may be causing anxiety. Any number of things can undermine her basic sense of control—a preschool class that's too rigid or advanced, a schedule that has too many structured activities and not enough time for free play, a personality clash between your child and her teacher, a family illness or divorce. Reducing the stress in your child's life can make a big difference in tantrum behavior.

You may also want to look more closely at your child's language development. "The preschool years are a period of rapid growth in both speech (how children pronounce words) and language (how they use words to communicate)," says Karen Johnson, M.S.ed., a speech-language pathologist with the South Windsor Public School System, in Connecticut. "Delays in either area can cause the kind of intense frustration that leads to tantrums."

For example, a child with articulation (pronunciation) problems may not be readily understood by playmates or adults. While the child's comprehension, vocabulary, and communicative intent may be intact, he may have problems clearly expressing his needs and/or wants. If language skills are lagging (or hearing is impaired), the child may have trouble understanding what adults expect of him, or asking that all-important preschool question: why? These situations, too, can cause intense frustration.

"I know that language delay was a major cause of tantrums with my son, Sam," says Wendy White-Hensen, a mother of two. "He didn't talk at all—except to say no—until he was about 3½. When he wanted something, he'd have to point and point until I could figure out what it was. He couldn't just tell me. It was so frustrating—for both of us."

According to Johnson, you should consult a pediatrician or speech-language pathologist if, between ages 3 and 4, your child:

- Does not have a vocabulary of at least 500 words
- Cannot use two-to four-word sentences
- Cannot be understood clearly by her peers or other people outside the immediate-family circle (by age 4, a child should be intelligible, or understood, 90 percent of the time)
- Shows a great deal of frustration when trying to communicate
- Has trouble understanding and following verbal directions with two or three steps
- Has trouble asking and answering questions
- Has had a history of chronic ear infections

Any one or a combination of the above conditions could signal problems.

Aside from language delays and the other triggers already mentioned, there are a couple more things that can ignite a tantrum at these ages. One is the very normal desire to test one's parents. As Dr. Peter Williamson points out, "Kids are like little scientists. They are constantly developing hypotheses, testing them out, and then evaluating and acting on their results." From a preschooler's point of view, throwing a tantrum is not so much a way to show defiance as a way to figure out what an adult really means or intends to do. You can almost hear a kid this age thinking, "If I throw a tantrum in this store, will Mommy buy me a cookie?"; "If I cry really loud, will I still have to go to bed?"; "If I hold my breath or shout this word, what will Daddy do?"

Another possibility is that your child is deliberately trying to manipulate you. She may have learned, during the terrible twos, that whenever she screams and shouts, the adults around her jump and do; or she may want something so badly that she'll try anything— even a dramatic display of wailing—to change your mind. From the outside, manipulative tantrums look very similar to those caused by loss of control. There are, however, a couple of key questions you can ask to help you discern between the two:

1. *Is there one specific, easily identifiable thing my child hopes to gain from this tantrum?* If the tantrum trigger is obvious (your child wants that cookie or toy, for instance) rather than general or obscure (she's overtired; she missed lunch; she just all of a sudden started screaming), manipulation is probably the goal. You may even find yourself thinking, "No way; I'm not giving in," when a manipulative tantrum occurs (as opposed to the usual "Now what's wrong?").

2. *Does my child seem totally engulfed by her rage— like she just can't help it?* If so, she's probably not just trying to manipulate you: she's honestly out of control. As Stanley Turecki, M.D., child psychiatrist and director of the Difficult Child Center in New York City, points out, "Manipulative tantrums tend to be less intense than those that occur when

a child is truly out of control. They have more of a conscious, planned quality."

The reason it's important to know the difference between uncontrolled outbursts (or temperamental tantrums) and manipulative tantrums is that each requires a slightly different response. "With the former," says Dr. Turecki, "you can afford to be kind and sympathetic, since your child really can't help himself. You may even want to give him a hug, or say something like, 'I know this is tough for you; I'll help you to bring it to an end.' With a manipulative tantrum, however, your attitude should be very firm, as in 'There's no way you're gonna get this, kid.'" (Chapter Five goes into more detail on how you should react to tantrums.)

Keep in mind, however, that being firm still does not mean getting angry with your child, or acting mean when tantrums occur. Very often, a child who's throwing a tantrum to manipulate you will get so frustrated when you don't give in that the tantrum will shift from calculated to out of control.

Kelly Smith (not her real name) remembers this happening once, with her daughter Lillith: "We were in a department store buying clothes, and she found this beautiful 'church' dress she wanted, but it cost $80, and I had no intention of buying it. So, as I stood in line at the register to pay for our other clothes, she started crying and begging for the dress. When she saw I wasn't going to give in, she became even more upset. I was wearing an elastic-waist skirt, and she started pulling down on it—it practically came off me. Then she started smacking me with her hands. Somehow, I managed to stay calm, and just kept repeating

'Keep your hands to yourself.' As soon as the bill was paid, I dragged her out of the store as quickly as possible, sat her on a bench, and gave her time to pull herself together. The tantrum may have started out because she wanted to manipulate me into buying something, but it grew beyond the point where she could control it."

Even in preschool, and even when their initial intentions seem shady, kids shouldn't be punished for tantrums. Young children have strong emotions and desires, and they can't help it when they feel or want things. As a parent, you always have the right to say no, but you never have the right to expect that your "no" will not hurt your child's feelings. If her disappointment is so great she needs to cry, you need to give her the time to get over it.

As with toddler tantrums, you help the most at this stage when you learn to ignore outbursts, and concentrate instead on preventive actions. Now, however, you have a new and potent tool at your disposal: language. Little by little, you can give your child the words he needs to identify, understand, and express his powerful emotions. The more your child learns to say what he thinks, the less he'll need to act out.

BIG-KID TANTRUMS

AGE FLAG: 5 TO 6 YEARS

Despite what you may have heard or read, there is no such thing as being "too old" to throw a tantrum. Grade-school kids get stressed out and overwhelmed just like everybody else, and for some of them, throwing a tantrum still feels like the best (or only) way to cope.

In fact, many parents find that the first few weeks of kindergarten bring out the worst in their child—mainly because of all the pressure and stress this milestone brings (a long or longer school day, new classmates, a new teacher, new behavioral expectations, and so on).

"During his first week of kindergarten, my son Ross threw a huge tantrum every day in the car on the way home," says Trudy Eaton. "He'd seem fine when I picked him up, but within minutes of leaving the school parking lot he'd fall to pieces over some minor, totally unpredictable thing. Once, I happened to mention I had been to the store and bought his favorite chips, and he started screaming and kicking the dashboard—because I had gone to the store without him."

Even kids who haven't thrown tantrums for years—or who were never big tantrum-throwers in the toddler stage—may suddenly regress to kicking and screaming around age 5 or 6 if they feel especially stressed by new events in their life (the birth of a sibling, the death of a family member or pet, a chronic illness in someone at home, divorce, a new sibling, a bully at school, homework, a too-rigid teacher, and so forth).

"My oldest daughter, Alison, just sailed through the terrible twos," recalls Lynn North (not her real name). "I can't remember one major tantrum. But then around age 5, she suddenly started throwing them. I think it was the combination of having, first, a new sibling to contend with, and then a longer day at school. The stress just got to her, and she needed a way to blow off steam."

First grade can also be a particularly stressful year. "While the peak period for temper tantrums is between 15 and 36 months, there's often another peak at around age 6," notes Barbara Howard, M.D., assistant clinical professor of pediatrics at Duke University Medical Center in Durham, North Carolina. "Like the earlier stage, this is a time when kids are really stretching themselves developmentally."

The stretching comes in different areas, however, and big-kid tantrums look and sound a little different than those of the toddler variety. While 2-year-olds will act out their anger, for instance, older kids will verbalize it: "I hate you!" they may yell. "You're the worst mother (or father) in the whole world." You may even hear swearing or gruesome threats: "If you don't buy this for me, I'm going to chop your head off and throw you away." Also, rather than flail blindly about, an older child may deliberately break things or hurt a sibling to emphasize his rage.

Another major difference can be seen in tantrum triggers. Older kids tend to be less concerned with issues like independence and separation from adults and more easily frustrated by fears about their own competency or by competition with other kids. At this stage, they have a clearer understanding of what adults expect of them (to sit still and listen in school, for instance, or to stand in line and wait their turn), but they still often lack the ability to comply (they just can't sit still or they feel too excited to stand in line).

Their social awareness is also much sharper. This is the age when kids begin to measure themselves carefully against their classmates and other peers ("She's good at drawing, but I'm better in math"; "He can kick really well, but I run faster"). While this ongoing analysis can lead to pride over accomplishments, it can also trigger feelings of shame and embarrassment if the child takes what he sees as his shortcomings too seriously. This is because 5-and 6-year-olds don't just make comparisons (for example, "Sally got a cat sticker from the teacher, and I got a dog"), they try to attach meaning to disappointing or frustrating events ("She knows cats are better than dogs, so that must mean she likes Sally better"). As wild as some of their interpretations may seem to us, they feel very real to them and can affect their behavior.

"With all of these changes and pressures, you shouldn't be too surprised or worried if your grade-school child throws an occasional tantrum, or goes through a brief period of tantrum behavior after a major transition," says Karen Buchanan, a parent educator for Project Enlightenment, an early-intervention program of the Wake County Public School System, based in Raleigh, North Carolina. "However, if tantrums are frequent or intense at this point, they should be evaluated more closely."

The American Academy of Pediatrics agrees. It recommends consultation with a physician if your child's tantrums significantly worsen after age 4 and/or she does any of the following:

• Injures herself or others during tantrums
• Destroys things during tantrums
• Has frequent nightmares
• Loses toilet-training skills
• Suffers frequent headaches or stomachaches
• Clings to you

- Displays a persistent negative
  esteem

A physical problem—such as hearing
or a chronic illness—may lie behind the ta
they may be an early sign of emotional proble   r a
symptom of language delay. Treating the underlying
problem will usually reduce or eliminate the tantrums.

If an evaluation indicates no medical or emotional
concerns, treatment is up to you. At this age, tantrums
should not be viewed as a normal step in development,
but as an indication of need: your child's need to learn
better ways of behaving.

Fortunately, there are several steps you can take
to prevent tantrum behavior, and minimize its impact
whenever it occurs (see Chapters Four and Five). The
key is not to waste your time and energy worrying
about what's wrong with your child or what you've
done to ruin him, but to act. As you'll learn when you
read through the rest of this book, when it comes to
tantrums, nature and nurture are inextricably inter-
twined—and both can be coaxed into positive growth.

❧ TWO

The Role of Temperament

With his round brown eyes and wide, bright smile, 3-year-old Justin is everyone's favorite kid. From the moment he was born, he's been easy-going. He makes friends quickly, plays well with other children, and hardly ever complains. He loves trying out new foods and activities, and adapts well to new situations. Now and then he'll throw a tantrum—but it's usually because he's tired or hungry, and his outbursts dissipate quickly.

Three-year-old Laura, a tiny brunette with intense blue eyes, won't crack a smile unless everything's perfect. She clings and whines in new situations, hates new clothes, and usually frowns when offered new foods. For her, tantrums are frequent and intense, and it takes a long time to calm her down.

Parents with kids like Justin usually feel pretty good

about themselves during the tantrum years. Their children rarely lose control, and when they do, it's fairly easy to get them back on track. Parents of children like Laura, however, often feel like failures. They never know when or where an outburst will happen, and nothing they do seems to help. They feel humiliated by their child's behavior, frustrated by their inability to stop the tantrums, and fearful that it's all their fault.

"At one point, when he was 4, my son Sam was throwing at least two major tantrums a day," recalls Wendy White-Hensen. "People stopped inviting him to come over and play and, I suspect, stopped inviting us over as a family. I felt isolated, angry, and resentful. I was convinced that my kid was far worse than anyone else's and that somehow I was to blame."

Not long ago, many child "experts" would have agreed. As late as the 1950s, the mental health field was dominated by a "blame the mother" ideology that linked poor parenting to everything from simple behavior disorders to adolescent delinquency, serious psychiatric disturbance, and even asthma. It was widely believed that in the earliest years of a child's life, a parent's least little remark or action could undermine future happiness.

Aside from causing widespread guilt among mothers, this ideology left many questions unanswered. For instance, if nurturing were so crucial, why was it that no one set of discipline techniques was effective with all kids? And why did some perfectly normal, laid-back parents produce dramatic, hot-tempered children, while some seriously disturbed parents produced calm, healthy ones? And what about siblings? So many of them seemed to display opposite behavioral traits.

Among those who wanted answers were Stella Chess, M.D., and Alexander Thomas, M.D., psychiatrists at New York University Medical Center. Based on observations of their own children, their friends' children, and the children in their practice, they were convinced that babies are born with innate differences in how they behave and react to the world around them. Some will startle at the slightest sound, for instance, while others can sleep soundly with the TV blaring and the vacuum on. They suspected that these differences in temperament persist through childhood, and are just as important as the parents' influence in shaping an individual's development.

In 1956, the two launched a longitudinal study (still ongoing) of 133 New York infants that eventually broke the existing mold. By identifying specific temperamental traits and following their effects from infancy through young adulthood, they were able to demonstrate that parents aren't always to blame for their kids' behavior.

Now, many experts agree that all of us are born with an inherited physiological bias—or temperament— that affects not only how we feel, react to things, and learn, but how other people react to us. This does not mean that our personality, intelligence, talent, physical abilities, or motivation are fixed at birth. It merely means that each of us has an inborn bias toward certain styles of behavior.

What Temperament Is

How a child:

* Feels when stressed or stimulated
* Is inclined to act in different circumstances
* Reacts to environments, events, and people
* Learns

What Temperament Is Not

An indication of your child's:

* Personality
* Intelligence
* Physical appearance
* Talent
* Physical ability
* Motivation
* Chance for future success

"Temperament is the how of behavior, not the why," explains Dr. Turecki, a coauthor of *The Difficult Child*. "The key question is not 'Why does my child behave that way when he doesn't get what he wants?' but 'When my child doesn't get what he wants, how does he express his displeasure?' Does he pout? Does he whine or complain? Does he kick and scream?"

In other words, the propensity for one child to feel like wailing for half an hour when his cookie breaks, while another may cry softly for a minute and then walk away, is not a function of poor parenting or an unhealthy environment. It is the result of an inherited physiological bias whose roots are still not completely understood.

"We have found that even in infancy, children vary considerably in how they respond to frustration," says Mary Rothbart, Ph.D., professor of psychology at the University of Oregon in Eugene. "In addition, tests have shown that certain behaviors identified at age 10 months are predictive of anger and aggression up to 7 years later."

While you can (and, in the case of temper tantrums, should) influence your child's behavior (how she acts), you cannot change her inborn temperament (how she feels like acting). But just knowing that certain aspects of who your child is are beyond your control can be extremely helpful. For one thing, it can alleviate a great deal of guilt if you have a child like Laura. For another, it can give you insight into what your child needs to learn, and how best to teach it.

"Children not only show differences in their emotional sensitivity and responsiveness, they also vary in how they think about and organize their experiences, tolerate external stimulation, and respond to rewards and punishments," says Dr. Williamson. While one kid with a volatile temper may show improvement if you talk to him in a soft voice and do lots of hugging, another may need firm, no-nonsense limits before he'll change a behavior.

Even with discipline, children respond in different ways. Studies show that infants who exhibit an "uninhibited temperament" (highly relaxed and sociable, not overly sensitive to outside stimulations) at age 3 to 5 months tend to be less intimidated and influenced by parental disapproval in later childhood than those with "inhibited" temperaments (who cried a lot in infancy, and were easily aroused by stimulation), according to Jerome Kagan, Ph.D., professor of psychology at Harvard University in Cambridge, Massachusetts.

What all this boils down to is this: parents of children like Justin aren't necessarily better parents—they just have easier kids. Even if your child is a Laura, you can reduce tantrums and make life more pleasant for both of you by learning to work with—rather than against—your child's temperament.

As Patricia Sutter found, "From the moment they were born, my twins, Matthew and Michael, were very different. Matthew was more relaxed and easy-going—you could take him anywhere. Michael, however, was very sensitive to stimulation, more active, and very particular about things. As a toddler, he was more easily frustrated than Matthew, had a much harder time making transitions, and threw more tantrums.

"I found that the better I got at understanding the differences between the two boys and planning ahead to alleviate frustration for Michael, the fewer tantrums we saw. Now I know that Michael just needs a little more time and patience before he can handle certain things—but he's still every bit as wonderful as his brother."

IDENTIFYING TEMPERAMENT

At some level, most parents, like Patricia, are aware of at least a few of their kids' main temperamental traits. We've all made excuses for our children's erratic behaviors ("Oh, she's just high-strung," or "He's hot-tempered and oversensitive"). And most of us are guilty of either comparing our kids ("He's so finicky, but she'll eat anything"; "She's the student, he's the clown"; "She's my athlete, he's my artist"), or blaming our spouse for any less-than-perfect qualities we see (as in "She's just like your crazy Aunt Beatrice" or "He obviously got his temper from your side of the family").

Drs. Chess and Thomas introduced a more scientific approach. As part of their longitudinal study, they needed a way to identify, define, and rate different categories of temperament, so they could follow them over the long term. With the help of Herbert Birch, M.D., then a behavioral scientist at Albert Einstein Medical Center in the Bronx, New York, they eventually settled on nine distinct traits, and a rating scale ranging from high to low (to represent differences within the wide range of normal behavior).

While neither definitive nor foolproof (other scientists have subsequently developed different models), the Chess–Thomas categories still provide a viable structure for examining your child's temperament. As you read through each one and fill out the worksheet on page 35, try to think about how your child has behaved since birth. The following examples of "high" and "low" behaviors will help you see how the different traits may evolve, from infancy through preschool. (If a particular behavior started recently, not soon after birth, it's probably not temperamentally based.)

———————————— ✳ ————————————

Worksheet: Defining Your Child's Temperament

Based on how your child has behaved since birth, how would you rate her on the following temperamental traits? (For help with ratings, refer to the examples on pages 36 to 39).

	Low	Medium	High
Activity level	_____	_____	_____
Regularity	_____	_____	_____
Approach	_____	_____	_____
Withdrawal	_____	_____	_____
Adaptability	_____	_____	_____
Sensory threshold	_____	_____	_____
Intensity	_____	_____	_____
Distractibility	_____	_____	_____
Persistence/attention span	_____	_____	_____
Quality of mood	_____ Positive _____ Negative		

———————————— ✳ ————————————

Temperament Traits

The Chess–Thomas temperament categories are as follows:

1. *Activity Level*—the amount of physical movement a child performs, and the proportion of active to inactive periods per day. Examples:

    High activity—a baby who squirms and splashes vigorously at bathtime, and later becomes a preschooler who's always running, never resting

    Low activity—a baby who can turn over, but rarely does; a preschooler who prefers books and puzzles to playgrounds and parties

2. *Regularity (or Rhythmicity)*—the predictability (or unpredictability) of a child's daily patterns of eating, sleeping, and defecating. Examples:

    High regularity—a baby who has a bowel movement every day after breakfast; a preschooler whose biggest meal is always lunch

    Low regularity—an infant who wakes six times one night and four times the next; a preschooler who's hungry at different times every day

3. *Approach/Withdrawal*—how a child initially responds to a new situation, food, toy, person, place, or other stimulus. Examples:

High approach—a baby who loves to smile at strangers; a preschooler who plunges right in at a new school

High withdrawal—a baby who always spits out new foods; a preschooler who takes weeks to warm up to a new play group

4. *Adaptability*—how easily a child adapts to a new or altered situation over the long term. Examples:

High adaptability—a baby who gobbles down a new food after only one or two introductions; a preschooler who falls asleep easily in her own bed the night of moving to a new home

Low adaptability—a baby who screams and struggles every time you put her in her snowsuit; a preschooler who takes months to feel comfortable in a new classroom

5. *Sensory Threshold*—the point at which any given stimulus will evoke a response from the child. Examples:

High threshold—a baby who bumps her head but just keeps on crawling; a preschooler who will eat anything, no matter what its smell or texture

Low threshold—an infant who startles at the slightest sound; a preschooler who refuses to wear new clothes because they're too stiff and itchy

6. *Intensity*—how forcefully a child expresses his reactions, whether positive or negative. Examples:

> *High intensity*—A baby whose cry is always loud
> and piercing; a preschooler whose laughter
> verges on hysteria

> *Low intensity*—a baby who expresses displea-
> sure by fussing, not crying; a preschooler who
> smiles quietly when she gets a new toy she loves

7. *Distractibility*—how well the child can pay attention, and how easily she is distracted. Examples:

> *High distractibility*—A baby who will stop nurs-
> ing if someone walks by, and won't resume until
> the person leaves the room; a preschooler who
> asks for a special kind of cookie—but easily ac-
> cepts a substitute if you can't find the type she
> wants

> *Low distractibility*—an infant who won't stop
> crying—even if you offer an interesting new
> toy—when she's waiting for a bottle; a pre-
> schooler who refuses to eat a lollipop because
> you gave him an orange one and he wanted red

8. *Persistence/Attention Span*—the length of time a
child can stay engaged with a particular object or
activity, even in the face of obstacles and difficulties. Examples:

> *High persistence/long attention span*—a baby
> who keeps crawling back to an electrical outlet

you pulled her away from, or who plays content-
edly for long periods with the same toy; a preschooler who spends an hour or so building a
fort with blocks

Low persistence/short attention span—a baby
who only plays for a few minutes with any one
toy; a preschooler who asks you to teach him to
draw a horse, but loses interest after the first try

9. *Quality of Mood*—the child's basic disposition. Examples:

Positive mood—a baby who smiles and coos
when she sees her bottle; a preschooler who
can't wait to show everyone her latest creation

Negative mood—a baby who always seems to be
crying, whining, or fussing; a preschooler who
constantly complains about the other kids in
his class

While there are many more examples and variations
for each of these categories, there is no evidence that
any of the traits listed are inherently "good" or "bad."
How each one is perceived depends on its context,
says Dr. Chess. "For example, high persistence may
come in handy when you want your child to clean her
room or finish an art project," she explains, "but it
may fuel a tantrum when you insist that your child put
down a toy and come to dinner."

Also, just as every child has a unique behavior style,
every household has its own personality. What's
viewed as a problem in one may be seen as a bonus in

another. If you and your spouse are the kind of parents who consider a day at an art museum the perfect outing, for instance, you may have trouble seeing positive qualities in a high-activity, high-approach child, who always wants to touch, climb, run, and jump on things. If your interests lie more in outdoor sports and new adventures, you'd probably think that same child was nearly perfect.

Even within the same family, one parent may have a better "fit" with a child than the other. This is because parents, too, have temperamental biases that predispose them to certain behavioral preferences. A low-activity parent who likes to read or work on long sit-down projects might have an especially difficult time dealing with a short-attention span child who can't sit still for long and is constantly craving something new. That same child may feel far less frustrated—and throw fewer tantrums—around another parent (or other caregiver) who's highly active and distractible, and who thrives on novelty and adventure.

Opposites don't always irritate, of course. Sometimes they create a perfect fit. As Dr. Turecki points out, a calm, low-key parent may enjoy or admire a child who's more active or intense than they are, and be patient enough to tolerate frequent tantrums.

"I know my son Ross saves up his worst tantrums for me," says Trudy Eaton. "In fact, a lot of his more volatile traits come from me. I am much more likely to react to things than my husband, who never gets ruffled by anything. He is always totally calm and consistent."

Temperament traits may also be viewed differently

at different stages of your child's development. As Drs. Chess and Thomas point out in their book, *Know Your Child: An Authoritative Guide for Today's Parents,* "High distractibility may be an advantage in a young child, making it easier for the parents to divert her from potentially dangerous activities. At a later age, however, this same distractibility may make her forget prearranged appointments or activities, as she gets diverted on the way home or on the way downstairs to breakfast."

The point is, none of these traits means that your child is "good" or "bad." How you rate him on the worksheet will have as much to do with your own temperamental biases and stress level (not to mention your exposure to other young children) as it has with your child's actual behavior.

In fact, it may be worth it to get outside help in identifying your child's temperament. As Dr. Kagan points out, "When you love someone, it's not always easy to detect temperamental traits—you have too many blind spots." To get a clearer picture, enlist the help of an unbiased observer (a wise friend, a trusted caregiver, a level-headed grandparent). Ask that person to fill out the worksheet, too, and then compare notes. You may also want to take some time to identify a few of your own temperamental biases. The list on pages 42 to 44 offers examples of how temperament traits can translate into adult behavior. By comparing your major characteristics with your child's, you may be able to pinpoint some conflicting traits that make trantrums more likely when the two of you are together.

✳

Adult Temperament Traits

1. *Activity Level*

    High activity—you're always on the go; you never want to sit home on the weekends; you remain physically active throughout life.

    Low activity—your favorite activity is sitting in front of the TV or curling up with a good book.

2. *Regularity (or Rhythmicity)*

    High regularity—you eat the same thing for breakfast every day and go to sleep at the same time every night.

    Low regularity—you often skip meals with no ill effects, and you never know when you're going to feel tired enough to go to sleep.

3. *Approach/Withdrawal*

    High approach—you love meeting new people and trying new things.

    High withdrawal—you dread situations that involve new places, activities, or food.

4. *Adaptability*

    High adaptability—when you make a new move or big change, you throw yourself into your new life.

Low adaptability—it takes you a long time to accept and see the good in a new move or other life change.

5. Sensory Threshold

High threshold—clutter, noise, and odors do not interfere with your ability to work or relax.

Low threshold—you are easily bothered by sights, sounds, and odors that others ignore.

6. Intensity

High intensity—you laugh loudly, get upset easily, and feel comfortable expressing your opinions strongly.

Low intensity—you are content to listen rather than speak, even when you don't agree with others; you are easy-going and optimistic even when things go wrong.

7. Distractibility

High distractibility—you can switch gears easily; you may have trouble meeting deadlines because you get interested in other things.

Low distractibility—once you've started a task or project, you don't let up until it's finished.

8. *Persistence/Attention Span*

> *High persistence/long attention span*—once you get interested in something, you can focus on it for long periods of time.

> *Low persistence/short attention span*—you like to take frequent breaks when involved in any project or activity.

9. *Quality of Mood*

> *Positive mood*—you're always smiling, laughing, and seeing the good side of life.

> *Negative mood*—you often feel blue, and expect the worst of most situations.

Temperament Types

The worksheet in this chapter can be useful in two distinct ways: (1) you can look at it as a chart, and try to determine whether there is a pattern to how you rated your child's temperamental characteristics (for example, do most of your checks fall into one of the three columns?); or (2) you can use it to identify individual characteristics that may trigger or intensify tantrums.

The first approach won't work for everyone, since more than a third of children do not show a distinct pattern of temperament traits. However, for those who do, identifying how the traits cluster can clue you in on what to expect in terms of tantrum behavior.

"EASY" KIDS

If most of your responses fall along the "medium" column, chances are you have a fairly laid-back child. Drs. Chess and Thomas found that about 40 percent of the children they studied had a combination of temperamental attributes that made them "easy" to parent. Their predominant traits were:

- Regular biological functions (medium rhythmicity)
- A generally positive approach to most—though not all—new situations and people (medium approach)
- Easy adaptability to most changes (medium adaptability)
- A mild or moderately intense mood that was mostly positive

"This is the kind of kid you can take anywhere," says Dr. Chess, "because he makes you look like a great parent. He doesn't misbehave much, and when he does, he adapts easily to the prevailing child-care techniques."

"Easy" children do have temper tantrums, but they tend to be infrequent and relatively mild, she adds. "When they occur, they usually mean that something drastic has happened, and you need to find out what it is. Often, just identifying the cause of the tantrum and eliminating or avoiding the trigger will quickly improve behavior."

"DIFFICULT" KIDS

If you notice a preponderance of checks along the "low" and/or "high" columns, you can be sure of something you've probably already suspected: your child is "difficult" to parent—or at least more challenging than average. Drs. Chess and Thomas found that about 10 percent of their study participants fell into this category. These kids are normal, and in some cases very intelligent, but they tend to:

- Be highly irregular in their eating, sleeping, and defecating habits (low rhythmicity)
- Resist new situations, foods, and people (high withdrawal)
- Adapt slowly to change (low adaptability)
- Have moods that are predominantly negative (negative mood)
- Feel easily provoked (high intensity)
- Be difficult to distract (low distractibility)

Dr. Turecki, who has expanded the clinical definition of *difficult* to encompass all nine categories of temperament, estimates that up to 20 percent of all American children under the age of 6 are "temperamentally difficult" or "hard to raise."

Though "difficult" children are not by definition "tantrum-prone," they do tend to get upset more easily, and their outbursts are often louder, more prolonged, and more dramatic than average. However, the label *difficult* does not mean your child is abnormal in any way. It's just a way of categorizing an extreme group of temperamental traits. As Dr. Chess explains:

"We coined this term because we found in our study that parents with this type of child had special difficulties in their management. But what we refer to as 'temperamentally difficult' may or may not coincide with a parent's label of 'a difficult child to manage.' Some parents can adapt easily to such a child; others will label a child 'difficult' for other reasons, such as low sensory threshold, high distractibility, or extreme persistence."

Even researchers have different ideas about what makes a child "difficult" or prone to tantrum. Dr. Rothbart, for example, has found a correlation between later anger and children who are by temperament:

- Highly active and goal oriented (even at a young age, they seem to know exactly what they want)
- Easily frustrated (they tend to react negatively when their goals are blocked)

The important thing is not to get caught up in labeling your child, but to understand that your kid may be more challenging, more willful, more stubborn, more sensitive, or more active than others—through no fault of yours or his—and he may throw tantrums more easily, dramatically, and intensely than others—because he can't help it.

"Some children, from infancy onward, are just more emotionally reactive than others," says Dr. Williamson. "They have a harder time regulating their feelings and behavior, and are more likely to have prolonged and intense emotional reactions when they don't get their way."

Learning this can be incredibly liberating. As one parent confides, "I used to think there was something wrong with me, because it always took my daughter 20 or 30 minutes to finish a tantrum, while other kids her age seemed to recover in a minute or two. But then I had a second child, who from the moment of birth was much more laid back and easy. She threw far fewer tantrums to begin with, and got over the ones she did throw much more quickly—even though I reacted to the tantrums in the exact same way. I finally understood that I wasn't the problem; my older child is simply more sensitive and intense than a lot of other kids, and needs more patience and guidance in mastering self-control."

"Difficult" kids may be harder to raise, but they are not lost causes. In fact, very often, the traits that give them trouble in childhood propel them to success later on. "A high-intensity child who tends to be extremely loud and overdramatic when it comes to expressing her feelings," says Dr. Turecki, "could end up in a career where such energy and vitality are essential, or a low-threshold kid who's hypersensitive to touch, taste, smell, and sound could grow up to be a marvelous chef or an interior designer. What you now see as disadvantages in temperament could, in later life, become helpful."

Also, temperament may be inborn, but it is not permanent and unchanging. How you react to your child's "difficult" traits will either minimize or exaggerate her tantrums (for more on this, see Chapter Three). In addition, once your child starts mingling more with peers at school, she may have more incentive to acquire better control. "Given sufficient time and patient handling, temperamentally difficult children do adapt well," stresses Dr. Chess, "especially if the people and places in their world remain constant and caring."

"QUIET" KIDS

If your child has some "difficult" traits (checks in the "high" and "low" columns), but rates only "medium" in intensity, she may be what Drs. Chess and Thomas identified as "slow to warm up." These children tend to:

- Respond negatively to new situations and people (low approach)
- Adapt slowly to change (low adaptability)

You might even call them shy, but their biological rhythms are more regular (medium regularity) and their intensity level is much milder (medium intensity) than that of "difficult" children, so in general, they're easier to live with. According to Dr. Chess, approximately 15 percent of kids fall into this category.

Slow-to-warm-up children rarely explode in an all-out tantrum. Instead, when upset or frustrated (often because you've pushed them too far, too fast), they put up a mild fuss and then withdraw quietly. "Unfortunately," says Dr. Chess, "this type of kid doesn't make much noise, so it's easy to overlook her. There could be something dreadful bothering her, but you'd never know it because she doesn't show it."

Slow-to-warm-up kids need extra encouragement in expressing strong feelings; that may even mean silently applauding your child when a tantrum happens, and giving her plenty of emotional space to blow off steam. You still shouldn't give in to her outbursts, but you should take extra pains to let her know that her feelings are normal and can be expressed in safe, healthy ways.

OTHER KIDS

If your child does not fall neatly into any one of the above categories (some 35 percent don't), you may need to probe a little deeper to understand his temperamental style. He may have just a few strong traits that are a problem only when your life style or environment directly clashes with them (when a high-activity child is forced to sit still on an airplane, for instance, or a high-persistence kid isn't given sufficient time to play with a new toy before bedtime). Or you may find that during particularly stressful times, your child does better around one parent than another because of how their temperaments fit.

As you read through the next section and think about your child's temperament and behavior, keep in mind that your goal is not to label your child and accept your fate (as in "She's just difficult—there's nothing we can do about it!"), but to use your deeper knowledge of her temperament to minimize and manage temper outbursts (as in "She's always had a hard time paying attention, so when we really want her to do something, we need to minimize distractions").

TEMPERAMENT TRIGGERS

Even if your child does not fit into one of the Chess–Thomas categories, you may be able to better understand her tantrum habits by examining her specific temperamental traits. Look again at your completed worksheet and try to identify any extreme traits (those with "high" or "low" ratings) your child exhibits; then see if they play a role in the kinds of things that typically trigger tantrums. For example:

- A kid with low regularity who's hungry at different times every day may throw frequent tantrums either at the table (when he's not hungry, but feels forced to eat), or between meals (when he needs a snack, but can't have one because "it's not time yet"). Understanding that your child has irregular rhythms (and has had them since birth) can help you see that such tantrums are not deliberate attempts to con you into giving treats or to ruin everyone else's supper, but a sign that you are working against his temperament. You can reduce a good number of food-related outbursts just by making healthy snacks (fruit, crackers and cheese, raisins, yogurt, and so on) available to him whenever he's hungry, and not fussing too much over how much he eats—or doesn't eat—during dinner. He should still come to the table with everyone else, but he shouldn't be forced to clean his plate.

- A child who constantly explodes when you ask her to put on new clothes or put away her favorite pair of sweatpants may not be just annoyingly picky. She may have a low sensory threshold that makes her extra sensitive to the feel of stiff, new, or scratchy materials. Knowing this, you could reduce tantrums by making an extra effort to buy softer, all-cotton clothing for her, and washing anything new three or four times before she wears it.

· A child who frequently throws tantrums outside the house, especially when there are new people, new foods, or new settings involved, may also rate high on withdrawal. The reason he starts clinging to you and whining in these situations is not because he's "acting like a baby," but because he feels temperamentally overwhelmed. The solution is not to avoid all new things or to keep your child tucked safely away at home. Instead, you can try to ease his anxieties by taking extra time to explain beforehand what's going to happen in new situations and giving frequent warnings ("It will be time to pick up the toys in five minutes") before a change in activity is about to occur.

You will not be able to attribute every tantrum your child throws to her temperament, nor should you try. There are many other factors—including your behavior, environment, stress levels, and health—that affect temper outbursts. But as Dr. Turecki notes, "Any time you can link your child's tantrums to a difficult temperamental trait, you are in a much better position to know what to do about it, and you're far more likely to be sympathetic."

The importance of a sympathetic attitude should not be underestimated, especially if you have a "difficult" or tantrum-prone child: sympathy does not come easily when emotional outbursts are frequent and intense.

What does come easily is blame. "When parents don't understand the basis of a child's behavior, they tend to think it's deliberate," notes Dr. Turecki. "They assume the child is in full control, and assign power and motives to him that he doesn't possess. They then begin to see him as a powerful enemy, and think things like, 'He's just trying to humiliate me'; 'She's doing this to get back at me'; 'He has no willpower'; 'She's just selfish and ungrateful.' The next step, of course, is punishment."

Unfortunately, punishment is the worst response you can give when a child has lost control over an assault to his temperament. A shy child can't help it if he dissolves into tears when thrust into a room full of strangers; a highly persistent child can't handle it when a favorite toy is whisked out of his hands. Yelling, hitting, threatening, or hurting won't make your child's feelings go away. Instead, it'll add to his frustration and helplessness—and fuel more tantrums. On top of that, it will make your child see you as someone who's unfair and mean.

With sympathy ("I can see you're having a hard time with this"), you can put an outburst into perspective and react more appropriately. "If you can start with a basic acceptance of who your child is, you can go a long way in modifying his behavior," says Dr. Turecki.

Take the case of Gary, a bright, energetic 2-year-old, who had a habit of howling in the car: "Every time we took a trip, he'd be fine for about the first hour, and then he'd lose it," says his father, Roger Smith (not his real name). "He'd kick and scream until we either pulled over and took a break or he exhausted himself and fell asleep. It made me so angry because I felt like he was just doing it to get attention; he was too spoiled. So I'd either ignore his cries or yell at him."

It wasn't until Roger considered his son's behavioral history (his temperament!) that he was able to revise his own feelings and response. "One day, I started remembering what an active baby Gary was," Roger says. "He crawled and walked very early, and he was always on the go. Even today, he's much happier running loose on the playground than pent up in the house. That helped me realize that Gary wasn't trying to torture me in the car, he was trying to relieve himself of what seemed like torture to him—sitting restrained for long periods of time."

Realizing this has helped Gary's father reduce car tantrums. "Now when we take car trips," he notes, "I plan ahead to make those extra stops—and the ride is much smoother. If a tantrum happens, I feel more sympathy for Gary than anger, and I respond in a more civilized way."

Roger has the right idea. Being sensitive to your child's temperament and sympathetic to her feelings does not mean shielding her from every challenge or frustration in life. "It means finding a way to help your child live in harmony with the world around him," says Betty Smith Franklin, Ph.D., associate professor of psychology at Goucher College in Towson, Maryland. "If you can accept some of the limits of your child's temperament and learn to work around them," she adds, "you'll spend less time fighting and more time teaching—and modeling—self-control."

When Temperament Traits Cause Trouble

"Whenever your child's environment clashes with her temperament, a tantrum is likely," says Dr. Chess. Here are some examples:

The Trait	The Prime Time for Tantrums
Low regularity	When child feels forced to eat when not hungry, sleep when not sleepy, or use the potty when not ready
High withdrawal	When child goes to a new daycare or preschool, meets a new babysitter, goes to a birthday party, is forced to try a new activity or new foods
Low adaptability	When child is not allowed to eat her favorite food or wear her favorite clothes, gets a new decoration for her bedroom, has to move or change schools or caregivers, is confronted with a change in routine
Low distractibility	When child is expected to drop a toy and do something else quickly, can't get what he's asked for fast enough, decides he wants to do something and then finds out he can't
Low sensory threshold	When child is forced to wear new clothes before you've washed them, is trying to sleep and the TV is on downstairs, has to be in a room that smells "yucky," has to eat a food that looks or smells "yucky"

The Trait	The Prime Time for Tantrums
High activity	When child is expected to sit in a carseat for a long time, be quiet in a public place, not touch anything in a store, stay inside all day because it's raining
High persistence	When child decides he wants a blue ball and you try to hand him a red one, wants to play with the telephone cord, but you pull him away, is in the middle of coloring when it comes time for bed

TANTRUMS

❊ THREE

Parents, Pitfalls, and Problem Solving

As important as age, development, and temperament are, they don't tell the whole story when it comes to kids and tantrums. There is another, more controllable element that affects the frequency and intensity of children's outbursts: parents.

How you react to tantrums, handle discipline, and cope with your own frustrations and anger all impact your child's passage through the tantrum years. This doesn't mean you cause your child's tantrums, or that you're to blame if your kid has a penchant for dramatic outbursts. What it does mean is this: no matter what your child's stage of development or predisposition to tantrums, you can make a positive or negative difference. To achieve the former—and avoid the latter— you need to be aware of the various ways in which your own behavior affects your child's.

What follows is a look at four of the most common parent pitfalls—and what to do if you encounter them.

PITFALL #1: SETTING A BAD EXAMPLE

"The last thing I said to my husband before I left the house for work was, 'Don't forget to clean up the living room and set the table before I get home,'" recalls Marianne Best (not her real name), a nurse and mother of two. "We were having company over for dinner, and they were scheduled to arrive soon after I got out of work, so it was up to him to straighten up the kids' toys and have everything ready. By the time I got home, I was exhausted from working and nervous about getting the meal on the table on time. 'At least the house will be clean,' I told myself as I unlocked the front door. But the first thing I saw when I stepped inside was a sea of Legos; in the background, I could hear my husband laughing and roughhousing with the boys. I was furious. Before he could even explain, I started screaming: 'Look at this mess! How could you do this to me? Can't you ever take any responsibility for anything? Now the party is totally ruined. . . .' I went on and on—I even started throwing toys around—until I suddenly noticed my older son's face: It was white. I felt terrible, so I just stormed upstairs to cool down."

Even in adulthood, most people have moments like this, when their anger or frustration is so overwhelming they feel like they have to explode. When we're at our best, of course, we control such anger, or find healthy ways to release it and solve our dilemmas. But when we're tired, sick, worried or stressed, it's all too easy to lose control and yell at our kids, scream at our spouse, throw things, break things, or lash out and hit.

We may not think of such behavior as a tantrum,

but in reality that's exactly what it is: an uncontrolled outburst of emotion. Sometimes, it makes us feel better by helping us blow off steam, but other times, it causes us to do or say things we later regret.

Even if an adult-size tantrum brings us temporary relief, however, it is rarely good for our health over the long term, especially if outbursts are regularly aimed at a family member. Recent studies of fighting between married couples have shown that expressing anger in a hostile manner (blowing up, screaming, hurling insults, calling names, or blaming) increases blood pressure, lowers immunity, and speeds up the heart. But suppressing anger and rage causes similar ill effects. The healthiest way to fight, researchers say, is to express our anger—without being nasty.

Finding kinder ways to show anger is not only good for us, it's much better for those around us, especially our kids. Seeing an adult lose her temper is scary for a child, but it's also instructive. As Dr. Kagan of Harvard points out, "Parents are role models for their children. If you handle your own anger by acting aggressively toward others, yelling a lot, or being overly punitive or rejecting, your children will learn to do the same."

An occasional outburst, of course, is nothing to worry about (unless it leads to physical, verbal, or emotional abuse of someone else). Most people "lose it" now and then—especially when they have young children underfoot—and kids should know that. But they should also know when you think you've done something wrong. With a preschooler or older child, for example, you can verbally correct yourself by saying something like: "I was so angry that I threw the plate at the wall, but that was wrong. I should have hit my pillow or taken a long walk instead."

If your outbursts are frequent, however, no explanation in the world is going to convince your child that tantrums are inappropriate. As the old saying goes, actions speak louder than words; nine times out of 10, a kid will do as you do, not as you say.

Losing your temper has another tantrum-producing effect on your child—anxiety. "Seeing a parent out of control is frightening for a child," says James Windell, a Michigan-based psychotherapist, and author of *8 Weeks to a Well-Behaved Child.* "It makes her feel like the world is a dangerous place. This, in turn, fuels anxiety, which often leads to more tantrums."

Unfortunately, we aren't always aware of how we're acting when we're angry, or we feel so justified in being angry that we presume our kids can understand the difference between us blowing off steam and them throwing a tantrum. In most cases, they can't. Children do not have access to the complicated motivations behind adult behavior, and many blame themselves when a parent loses control.

----------------- ✳ -----------------

Tips for Taming Your Own Temper

Feeling intense anger is as normal for adults as it is for children. But throwing a tantrum is not. Here are some tips for taming your own temper—so you can better help your child tame hers:

1. Avoid known triggers. If, for instance, whining before breakfast is what really sets you off, ask your spouse

to take charge of the kids in the morning; if it's children who interrupt telephone calls, save phone use for nap times.

2. Adjust your expectations. Children are not miniature adults, and they don't have control over their words and actions the way grownups do. When your child's behavior begins to drive you crazy, try to see it from a kid's perspective, rather than an adult's. Find out what other children her age are doing. Above all, don't be afraid to acknowledge your child's right to want things—even if he can't have them.

3. Walk away. When you feel like you're about to explode, leave the room and try to cool down before you react. Tell the person at whom you're angry what you're doing: "I'm so angry that (such and such happened) that I'm leaving the room for a while to cool down." Then take a brisk walk, wash the dishes, weed the garden, punch a pillow—anything that helps you diffuse your pent-up energy and emotions—before you say or do something you may later regret. If you think walking away will make your child feel as though he's being abandoned, try this instead: take a deep breath and count to 10 before you say anything, or repeat to yourself a soothing phrase: "This is just a stage; it soon will pass."

4. Focus on the facts. If you find yourself thinking things like, "He's just trying to get back at me for not letting him play outside" or "She wants me to get angry and explode," force yourself to stop. Focus on the facts—what the person at whom you're angry did—rather than what you suspect his motives were.

5. Avoid blaming. Rather than pin your angry feelings on another person ("I wouldn't have exploded if you hadn't said that"), think about what it is that you're

most upset about, and why this particular thing angers you ("I hate it when people say [this particular thing] because it makes me feel [this particular way]).

6. Look at the bright side. If you can find a way to let humor reduce tension (picturing what your child would look like 20 years from now with spaghetti in her hair), use it to help you refocus and calm down.

7. Call a friend. Talking to someone you trust can help diffuse your anger and give you a new outlook.

A good way to find out what kind of example you're setting for your child is to keep a record of how you react to anger and frustration over the course of a few days or a week. Then, review what you've written, and pretend you're reading about your child's behavior. Does it seem acceptable to you? If not, you can be sure you need to change your ways.

Another way to discover your impact on others is to ask a trusted friend, your spouse, or another family member to describe what happens when you get really mad or frustrated, and how your behavior makes them feel. If others see your behavior as reasonable, your children will benefit by seeing you handle frustrating situations. If you frighten or embarrass your family and friends, however, you'll need to change your coping strategy (for more ideas, see Tips for Taming Your Own Temper on page 60). Remember, if you're not willing to change, you can't expect your child to.

PITFALL #2: LASHING OUT

"It had been a long, rainy day, and I had been stuck inside the house—alone—with my active, tantrum-prone 3-year-old," recalls Linda King (not her real name), a mother of two. "By late afternoon, I was tired, out of patience, and too drained to think creatively in response to my son's outbursts. At one point, when I had to change his diaper, he just wouldn't stand still. He kept running away, and I had to pick him up while he was kicking and screaming. After a while, I finally snapped: I grabbed him, turned him over, and slapped him so hard on the bottom I could see my handprint. He didn't even cry at first—he just looked at me with these wide eyes. I immediately felt terrible—and was frightened by my own lack of control. I had never hit him before. It was awful. The next day, I called a child psychologist, and asked for help dealing with my son's tantrums."

No matter how much you love your child, at some point when he's throwing a tantrum, you'll probably feel the way this parent did: so angry and frustrated you'd gladly give him away. You may even momentarily hate your child or feel a resentment that's so intense you find yourself doing or saying things you'd never dream of in a saner moment—like slapping your child or screaming about how he's just "a selfish little brat."

Before you write yourself off as a failure at parenting, consider this: in a study by researchers at Iowa State University in Ames, almost two-thirds of fathers and three-quarters of mothers admitted that they lose their cool at least half the time when their kid does something they believe is wrong.

Tantrums are an easy trigger for parental anger because they fuel so many different emotions: bewilderment, embarrassment, anxiety, guilt, resentment, disappointment, and helplessness, to name a few. Plus, there's the sheer frustration of trying to make a child who can't stop crying calm down, and the ego-destroying blow of being repaid for your efforts with more intense crying, screaming, or complaining. As one mild-mannered New York father admits: "Sometimes, when my son has a prolonged tantrum, I reach a point where I think that the best—and possibly only—way to get him to stop would be to slap him really hard. I know that sounds terrible, and I'd never actually do it, but that's how his behavior makes me feel."

A mother from Connecticut confides: "When my daughter is having a tantrum and I try to help her, she just keeps getting madder and madder at me. That, of course, makes me madder and madder, and sometimes I get to the point where I just want to choke her."

Fantasies like this may sound horrifying, but they're also surprisingly common. As Nancy Samalin points out in her book *Love and Anger: The Parental Dilemma,* "The subject of anger almost always comes up when parents gather, and it's a subject that troubles them a great deal. They believe that good parents don't yell, much less shriek; loving parents don't seethe with resentment; mature adults never give in to uncontrolled rage."

Nothing could be further from the truth, she adds. "The greater our love, the greater, too, our capacity for feeling a full range of troubling emotions, including anger, resentment, and even rage. It is only natural that these strong emotions are sometimes expressed in our relationships with our children, for they are the people in whom we invest our greatest love, our most intense feelings, and our highest expectations."

Understanding that it's normal to have brief moments of intense negative feelings toward your child is important; acknowledging those feelings—as ugly as they are—often helps to disarm them. As Samalin points out, "Just talking about how you feel to an understanding, nonjudgmental person can bring you some relief." If you don't acknowledge your negative thoughts, they're bound to surface in indirect ways (via hurtful teasing, name-calling, nagging, or even harsh punishment).

Also, there's a big difference between *feeling* a negative emotion or *fantasizing* about a harmful action—and *acting* on either one. Your child will not be harmed if, in your anger, you secretly imagine dressing her up in her prettiest outfit and putting her up for sale. But if you threaten to do that or you hit her, call her names, withhold your love, tell her that she (rather than her behavior) is bad, or show other forms of open aggression, damage will be done. "This kind of venting, especially in the midst of a rage, should never be directed at your kids," says Samalin.

───────────── ✳ ─────────────

Anger and Abuse

Though intense feelings of anger and resentment toward a child pass through most parents at some point or another, frequent feelings of hatred, resentment, or disgust are not normal; nor is acting upon such feelings—especially if they cause you to inflict physical or emotional pain on your child. You need to seek professional help if you:

- Frequently feel that you hate your child
- Think your child is bad, evil, or unworthy of your love
- Find yourself verbally, physically, or emotionally abusing your child when you are angry
- Feel depressed at the thought of spending time alone with your child
- Can never think of anything nice to say to or about your child
- Are feeling depressed

During a tantrum, it may take extra effort to remember this, and to resist the impulse to *act* on your feelings. As James Windell points out, "When parents feel inadequate or stressed in the face of a problem behavior (like tantrums), they often resort to the punishments popular when they were kids: spanking, yelling, lecturing, criticizing, and threatening. They figure they turned out okay, so it won't harm their children."

Research has shown, however, that harsh discipline techniques can cause harm, and they rarely cure problem behaviors. They may stop misbehavior in the short term, but in the long run they increase defiance and lower self-esteem. "Kids who feel attacked—either physically or verbally—by their parents become more anxious and defensive, not less," adds Windell.

Susan Crockenberg, Ph.D., professor of psychology

at the University of Vermont, in Burlington, agrees. In her studies of young children, she's found that those with mothers who frequently express anger are more defiant and show less concern for others than their peers. "When a child feels attacked by a parent," she explains, "his natural inclination is to be defensive, to think: 'I'd better be careful and pay attention to my own needs.'"

There are a number of other very good reasons to resist lashing out at your child when he's having a tantrum:

1. You may not be able to control yourself. As soon as you act on an angry impulse to stop the tantrum, you run the risk of feeling even more frustrated when your child doesn't (because he can't) comply. This, in turn, may escalate your actions—from yelling to threatening to spanking to beating, for instance. If nothing else, it almost guarantees that you'll say something ridiculous, such as "If you don't stop crying over that cookie right now, you'll never get another one ever again" or "Shut up, or I'll throw every one of those toys in the trash." Such empty threats only teach your child that you can't control your temper, either. Plus, they undermine your future efforts at discipline by making your child think things such as "She doesn't really mean what she says" or "He'd never really do that."

2. It sends a message that strong feelings of anger and frustration are "bad" or "wrong." What kids need to learn, instead, is that strong emotions are normal and can be dealt with in a healthy way before they

cause harm. You teach this best when you learn to shift your focus away from how a tantrum makes you feel (as in "This kid is driving me nuts"), to what it says about your child ("This tantrum tells me Johnny needs more help learning how to wait his turn").

3. It doesn't teach positive alternatives. When you hit or yell at kids, the only lesson they learn is that big, powerful people can bully and hurt smaller people. You do not teach them better ways to behave, which is what they really need to know. As Kathy Merritt, M.D., assistant professor in the division of general pediatrics at Duke University in Durham, North Carolina, explains, "The real purpose of discipline is not to punish, but to teach kids how to behave in socially acceptable ways, and how to control normal emotions, like anger, frustration, and jealousy."

4. It lowers your child's self-esteem. "One of your most important goals as a parent is to help your child feel lovable and capable," says Dr. Barbara Howard. "Physical punishment not only doesn't do either of those things, it is disrespectful to the child, and it fuels feelings of fear and anger." It has also been linked to depression, alcoholism, and poor resilience to stress in later life. "Ninety-eight percent of kids can be managed without ever being hit," she adds.

5. It gives your child attention, which reinforces tantrum behavior. Children view any parental reaction—even nagging and screaming—as a form of attention, and there's nothing the average kid craves more. If he can't get enough of it by behaving (sit-

ting and playing quietly, for instance), he'll switch to misbehaving (whining and tantrums) just to catch your eye. You may find this hard to believe, but most kids would rather be spanked than ignored.

In fact, noticing a child when she's being "good" (instead of when she's misbehaving), is far more effective in changing negative behaviors than any form of punishment. It may not feel natural to notice and praise your child when she's sitting around behaving or controlling her temper (after all, she's doing what she's supposed to be doing, so why make a fuss?), but according to most experts, it works. If you ignore appropriate behavior, and then drop everything to respond to a tantrum, you set yourself up for future explosions: even a 2-year-old can figure out which behavior brings the better pay-off.

Again, as difficult as it is to remain calm during a tantrum, it's essential that you try. Before you act, remind yourself that lashing out will only bring you temporary relief; in the long run, it'll make you feel more guilty (for saying and doing things you know you shouldn't), and make your child more likely to have tantrums (because she's scared, angry, or anxious, is enjoying the negative attention, or is just copying you). It is not always easy to put a child first during tantrum situations, but part of being a good parent is learning to make the kinds of sacrifices that really count. Controlling your temper is one of the biggest and most important sacrifices you can make for your child.

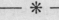

High Anxiety

Like adults, children are more likely to lose control when feeling stressed or anxious. You can help if you learn to avoid:

* Frequently pleading or bargaining with your child—so she won't think you have trouble setting and enforcing limits.

* Showing your own sadness or guilt when you take him to preschool or daycare—so he won't think there's a good reason for him to be upset, too.

* Making promises you can't (or don't intend) to keep—so you won't erode her sense of security and trust.

* Withholding your love or attention as punishment for misbehavior—so he won't feel insecure and go off to seek negative attention.

* Changing discipline decisions because you're afraid your child won't love you—so he won't be frightened by an inappropriate balance of power.

* Giving gifts and toys instead of time and attention—so he won't think you value things more than him.

PITFALL #3: STRUGGLING FOR POWER

"When Hugh was about 3 years old, we went through a stage where getting him to brush his teeth was a daily struggle," recalls Holly Hughes. "He'd throw a tantrum, and I'd practically have to pin him down to get his teeth cleaned. One night, when we were staying in a hotel before going to my sister's wedding, I just got fed up with the fight. I threw his toothbrush down and shouted at him, 'I don't care if your teeth fall out of your head. I'm not going to fight over this anymore.' He suddenly stopped his tantrum and just looked at me. A little later, my husband offered to help him brush, and he willingly complied. Since that night, toothbrushing has magically become a nonissue in our household."

In their never-ending quest for autonomy, young children (especially toddlers) are constantly testing their parents to find out who's really in charge. While they often feel comforted to know that there's an adult around to keep them from harm, they are just as often infuriated at the thought of someone bigger controlling them. When they feel especially thwarted in their desires or become locked in mortal combat with a stubborn adult, they use everything in their power— including tantrums—to win.

In fact, one of the easiest ways to arouse a young child's ire is to give a direct order. Research by Dr. Crockenberg shows that when a parent escalates a demand (going from "Pick up your toys," for example, to "You're not going outside until you pick up your toys"), the child's misbehavior mounts as well, until a tantrum or other negative action occurs. However, if the parent finds a way to restate her request in a less direct or even humorous way (as in "Who do you think could win a race to your toy box: your blocks or your dolls?) the child will usually back down and happily comply.

Words That Work

Here are some examples of how to make no sound like yes:

* "I can see how much you like that toy, but I'm not ready to buy it for you today. Why don't we put it on your wish list?"
* "Yes, you can have an apple and some juice—as soon as all of your toys are picked up."
* "I would be happy to get you another glass of milk—after you ask me in a nice tone of voice and say please."
* "It's a little too hot for your black shirt today, but you're welcome to choose between the red and the blue."

One of the quickest ways to eliminate a lot of temper tantrums, then, is to simply avoid engaging in power struggles with your child. I know, I know: this is far easier said than done. Outright defiance from someone who still wears diapers and sucks her thumb is difficult to ignore, as is whining from a child whose demands seem never-ending or absurd. As Dr. Lawrence Balter points out: "Kids can be incredibly fickle-minded and irrational. They may blow up at you for 'making them' break a toy when you weren't even in the same room, or throw a major tantrum over something that they won't even care about in a day or two."

Parental pride and wishful thinking also get in the way. Despite all evidence to the contrary, many parents persist in believing that their children will want to do as they ask, and will eagerly listen to their advice out of love and gratitude for the many sacrifices they've made on their behalf. When their kids then defy them (which is far more likely, more normal, and more healthy than constant obedience), they feel shocked, hurt, and angry. Then they worry that the child is becoming "spoiled," so they make up their mind to "teach her who's boss."

Of course, this rarely works. "When kids and parents lock horns over who's in control, one of two things usually happens," says Dr. Williamson. "Either the kid wins, or the parent has to go to such extremes of enforcement that she feels rotten afterward."

In either case, a power struggle teaches your child one main concept: that you and he are on different teams, and if he wants his team to win, he'll have to fight to the bitter end to beat you. In the case of a preschooler or toddler, the "bitter end" is almost inevitably a tantrum.

This kind of competitive rift can—and should—be avoided. "You can't expect total compliance from a child, anyway," says Dr. Merritt. "That would be unhealthy. So you should pick your battles carefully."

While there are certain issues an adult should never back down on—especially those involving a child's safety, health, and well-being—there are numerous others that can be negotiated or reframed without spoiling a child. These are the issues that have more to do with style (personal preferences) than substance (health, safety, values). For example:

- Your child may want to wear mismatched clothes to preschool.

  You may feel it's your duty to make sure he looks

presentable, however; you may even worry about what other parents or his teachers will think if he shows up in a green plaid shirt and pink striped pants or in mismatched sneakers. So you put your foot down. Unfortunately, forcing him to wear what you want at a time when he's just exploring his own tastes and ideas is bound to cause the kind of frustration that leads directly to tantrums.

In contrast, letting him experiment with clothing may lead to some pretty funky outfits, but it won't hurt anyone, and it won't warp his development. It will give him a healthy sense of confidence and control. As he grows older, peer pressure will kick in, and he'll beg you to buy him what everyone else is wearing anyway. On a scale of one to 10, with 10 being "essential to health and well-being," this issue would rate about two—as in not worth the fight.

You could easily end the power struggle—and any related tantrums—just by letting your child wear whatever he wants. Or, if you really can't bear looking at a mismatched child, you could quietly buy shirts and pants that match, and let your child create his daily wardrobe from a color-coordinated selection. That way, your child will feel good because he still gets to choose, and you'll stay happy because no matter what the combination of the day, he'll always be matched.

• Your child may insist on going outdoors on a cool day with no coat on.

If you're like most parents, you probably think you should force your child to bundle up (so the neighbors won't suspect neglect). But if you do, you may be starting World War III. In the long run, there will be far fewer tantrums over this issue if you let your child experiment—and experience the natural consequences of her choice. Let her run outside without a coat. As soon as she feels how cold it really is, you can be sure she'll be back at the door begging for it; if she plays happily without the additional warmth, she probably didn't need the extra layer after all. In the meantime, you've avoided a needless power struggle and boosted your child's sense of control and confidence at the same time. (If you are leaving the house for the day, of course, bring along the extra coat, hat, and scarf for when she changes her mind. She won't learn the lesson better if you make her freeze to death.)

• Your kid may indicate that he is physically capable of using the potty, but refuse to do so.

You can either plead, cajole, bribe, or try to force him to use it (which rarely works, and gives him a good excuse for tantrums), or accept the fact that you have no real control over his bowel and bladder, and allow him to lead the way. The former strategy is bound to bring conflict without changing behavior, while the latter will put the control where it belongs: in this case, with the child. All normal children do, eventually, learn to use the potty. The worst that will happen by abdicating your control is that you may have to change diapers for a little longer than you'd like.

• Your child wants to brush her teeth after her bath, but you want her to brush them before.

If giving her a choice of when to brush will make her more likely to brush without a fight, by all means let her have her way. The important thing is not when she brushes, but the fact that she's learning to take responsibility for an important part of her daily hygiene.

- You've worked hard to create a beautiful, well-coordinated bedroom for your son, and he wants to spoil it by hanging up a huge poster of his favorite superheroes or gory monsters.

There's no accounting for taste with kids. But even if the adults who visit your son's room wince at his choice, you're better off letting him explore his own ideas of what's visually appealing than enforcing yours. In the long run, letting him personalize his private space will help him feel more valued, more in control, and more confident about expressing his own ideas.

There are many more examples. The point is, you increase tantrums when you allow minor disagreements to blossom into power struggles. You'll reduce them, however, if you can resist the impulse to assert your authority, and learn, instead, to (1) acknowledge your child's wants and desires (as insatiable as they may seem), and (2) find ways to make her feel she has a say in what happens to her (even when she really doesn't).

"Sometimes," says Dr. Crockenberg, "you have to settle for something close to compliance. The other night I was taking care of my 3-year-old grandson and I needed to give him a bath. He, of course, said, 'No bath.' So, I told him, again, it was a bath night, and he said, 'Give me 5 more minutes to play.' I could have just insisted he get into the tub immediately (and spent 5 more minutes arguing about it with him), but instead

I said, 'Okay. Five more minutes of play.' When the time was up, he took his bath without a fight. Even when the child doesn't have a choice, try to find some aspect of the situation he can control—and let him."

As Dr. Turecki observes: "You can never be wrong to be emotionally generous with your child." It also helps to be well informed about child development. If you know it's normal for a 2-year-old to eat with his fingers, or for a 4-year-old to whine, you'll be less likely to crack down on such behaviors or misinterpret them as willful defiance. This, in turn, will lower tantrum levels in your household. According to the American Academy of Pediatrics, children whose parents are overly strict and punitive tend to have more frequent and severe tantrums than children whose parents take a moderate approach.

Whenever you sense that you and your child are about to butt heads, take a minute to ask yourself:

- Am I expecting too much (or too little) from my child?
- Could I get what I want in a more clever or humorous way?

Never back down on reasonable requests (about crossing the street with an adult, for instance, or eating vegetables before dessert), but do be flexible when your child has a logical reason for changing your mind or simply needs to feel more in control. "Sometimes," says Dr. Merritt, "our kids learn more from a situation when we allow them to save face."

PITFALL #4: GIVING IN

"One day, my 3-year-old son, Alexander, came across a bag of toys that I had bought to have on hand for various special occasions," says Margot Adler. "Some were for him, and some were for other kids, but none of them was meant to be seen or opened by him that day. When he realized I wasn't going to let him have the toys, he began to cry. I was able to distract him for a while, but he went back to the place where the bag was three different times, and was crying and crying. I finally relented and gave him one toy from the bag. I'm not sure whether it was the right or wrong thing to do—but I did feel it was too hard a task for him to have patience and wait for the toy once he had already seen it. I should have hidden the presents more carefully."

Most of us have been in this same position all too often. Our child throws a fit (usually in public, or when we're too tired or stressed to think straight!) and, against our better judgment, we stop the fuss the easiest way we know how—by giving in. It buys us temporary peace, but according to the experts, it also usually guarantees that another temper tantrum soon will follow.

Just as being overly strict can trigger power struggles and tantrums, so, too, can being too lax with our children by appeasing tantrums, failing to set reasonable limits on behavior, pleading and bargaining with our kids, or being inconsistent in our reactions and discipline.

Five Good Reasons Not to Give In

1. It rewards your child for throwing the tantrum—and thus ensures future tantrums.
2. It tells your child that you don't have faith in her ability to control herself.
3. It encourages your child to use anger to manipulate people.
4. It doesn't teach healthy alternatives for expressing anger and handling disappointment.
5. It gives your child a scary sense of having power over you.

As much as they fight for control, most children secretly don't want too much power over us. They recognize their own inability to cope with many of life's challenges, and they desperately want an adult around who will ensure their safety and provide support and guidance. When we give in to a tantrum (as opposed to changing our mind after hearing a reasonable, logical, calmly stated request), we basically inform our kid that her violent and aggressive behavior is powerful enough to bend our will and make us yield to her desires. That kind of power can be frightening to a child.

But in many ways, it's also irresistible. Once a kid figures out that tantrums get him what he wants, he'll use that tool whenever and wherever possible. As Dr. Kagan observes: "When you give in to a tantrum or respond in an inconsistent manner, what you're really doing is rewarding the child for that behavior."

There are many reasons why parents fall prey to giving in or to being inconsistent in how they react to tantrums (acting harshly one time, ignoring it the next, for example.) One is that we're often too exhausted after a hard day's work to deal with a child who's out of control. We want—and need—peace and quiet, so we take the path of least resistance and let the child have her way.

As Henry Cunningham observes: "How I react to my kids' tantrums usually depends on the situation and my own condition. If I'm feeling calm and energetic, I can usually find a way to distract the child, so he can calm down quickly and move on to a new activity. But if I'm overly tired or hungry myself, I may lose control and shout or just give the kid what he wants. I hate to do that because I know it means more tantrums, but sometimes, I just can't help myself. I get tired, too!"

This isn't at all unusual. "It's easy, after a day full of hassles, to experience a child as being just one more hassle, one more person who wants to sap our strength," says Nancy Samalin. "We feel emotionally fragile and put upon. We long to have someone take care of us and soothe our emotions. Instead, we are required to take care of a child who might be exhausted and needy as well and who is acting unreasonable. This child can become the enemy in our battle to have a moment's peace."

Another reason well-meaning parents give in to tantrums is guilt. Parents who spend a great deal of time away from their children often try to compensate when they're together by keeping their child constantly happy. They give in to the child's demands because they're afraid that if they don't, the kid might get angry at them or decide not to love them anymore (a very unlikely event, by the way).

Then there's the fear of harming a child's psyche: "Many parents have become gun-shy about discipline because they're afraid of doing lasting damage," notes Dr. Williamson. "Part of their fear stems from the child-rearing theories of the 1950s, which said that punishment was bad for children. But back then, nobody made a distinction between reasonable discipline and harsh punishment. Harshness doesn't help children, but clarity (in rules and consequences) helps them a great deal. It teaches them what to expect, how to behave, and how to cope with life's many challenges."

"Most children are a lot tougher psychologically than their parents think," adds Dr. Williamson. "They have to be, to endure the bumps and bruises involved in normal growing up." In most cases, saying no to a child is not nearly as awful as the child would have you believe. Kids are supposed to ask and test and cajole and complain—it's part of their strategy for learning about the world. Think about the kind of person your child would be in adulthood if she never had a chance to challenge you or any other adult as a kid. (Does the word *robot* come to mind? It should!)

Even so, it's the parent's job to decide when to say yes and when to say no. Your child may not like to hear the word *no;* she may even act like the world has come to an abrupt and bitter end. But that doesn't mean she'll be traumatized for life. At some point, if the limits you set are reasonable, she'll understand that you have her best interests and safety at heart.

What really counts is not so much *when* you say no, but *how* you say it. If you can do it in a way that acknowledges your child's right to want something, and to be upset at not getting it (for example, "I know you really want dessert and that you feel sad for not getting it, but in this house, we eat our dinner before we eat our sweets"), you'll go a long way in avoiding tantrums.

Remember: kids need clear, fair limits; they want to understand what you expect of them and what will happen if they misbehave; they actually feel more secure when they know that you will follow through on what you say. Giving in to a tantrum undermines not only your authority, but your child's opportunity to learn important lessons—such as how to delay gratification, how to behave in public places, how to treat siblings, how to express anger, how to tell when Mom and Dad have had enough.

ABOVE ALL: CONSISTENCY COUNTS

There are many other things parents inadvertently do to frustrate their children and encourage temper tantrums. Most of them boil down to:

- Expecting more (or less) of your child than he's developmentally or temperamentally capable of
- Not being clear about your expectations (for example, when you say "Clean your room," you mean you want her to pick up the books and the dolls and the blocks, and put them where they belong)
- Not setting clear and reasonable limits on behavior

- Not enforcing the limits you set
- Not following up on the discipline promised

Whenever kids feel like they are on shaky ground—especially when they don't know what to expect or how you're going to react to something—they feel anxious and vulnerable and are more prone to have a tantrum. "Your ultimate success in changing your child's tantrum behavior depends on your consistency," adds Dr. Garber. "Perhaps the most important guideline to follow is this: mean what you say, say what you mean, and make sure everyone involved is saying the same thing."

✿ FOUR

A Pound of Prevention

Just as parents can inadvertently encourage temper tantrums, they can also actively discourage them— but not when a tantrum's in progress. The best time to work on managing temper tantrums is when nothing special is happening: you're feeling calm, your child is relaxed, and neither one of you is overtired or on edge. The reason for this is twofold:

1. Kids learn better when they aren't feeling out of control or defensive. Trying to teach a child a better way to behave when he's in the midst of a blowout is like expecting him to understand a movie that's been dubbed in a foreign language: he can see your lips move, but he can't comprehend a word you're saying. Most children are too overwhelmed during a tantrum to even think, never mind listen.

   Punishing or lecturing a child just after a tantrum

is over rarely works, either, because it shames the child and puts her on the defensive. Think of how you feel when someone accuses you of doing something wrong. Is your first impulse a desire to deny the wrongdoing or to place the blame elsewhere? It is for many children, and since kids aren't as skilled at controlling their impulses as adults are, they often do just that. They blurt out excuses—"I wasn't yelling. I was trying to make you hear me!" or "I wouldn't have thrown a tantrum if you hadn't made me miss my TV show"—just to avoid getting in trouble. This is not the kind of mindset that encourages learning.

Another problem with always reacting to tantrums is that it tends to promote an escalating cycle of negative interaction. Typically, the parent becomes so frustrated by the child's tantrums that the least little outburst triggers an immediate punishment. Rather than stop the behavior, however, the punishment makes the child feel more angry, anxious, and frustrated—and more prone to throw tantrums. As the tantrums continue, the parent's frustration and helplessness grow, and the punishments either become widely inconsistent (harsh one time and lax the next) or escalate (from yelling to spanking, for instance). The harsher and more inconsistent the parent's response, the more frequent the tantrums.

Eventually, both child and parent become locked in what Dr. Turecki calls a vicious circle of tantrums and punishment. "The child never knows you're serious about helping him because you're screaming and yelling all the time," he adds. Again: not conducive to learning.

2. Prevention is still the best medicine. Every time you help your child avoid a temper tantrum or master her emotions, you show her that you're on her side—that you want her to feel in control and confident. At the same time, you encourage her to believe that she can control her actions and emotions.

Tantrums, after all, can be habit forming: the more your child has them, the more likely he is to turn to them when he needs to communicate, complain, or blow off steam. If you can reduce them in sheer number, you not only make the habit less likely to happen, you buy yourself the kind of peace and quiet you need to teach your child self-control.

Preventive measures work best, however, when you present them with the kind of self-control you hope to teach. You need to find ways to talk to your child about tantrums without accusing, blaming, or threatening; to speak in a calm, matter-of-fact voice that shows you genuinely care and want to help. Like adults, children have a hard time listening and learning when they don't feel respected and safe.

You also need to tailor your approach to your child's age, development, and temperament. Toddlers, for example, can't process verbal information the way 4-and 5-year-olds can, and older children need more specific rules and consequences to guide their behavior. Also, children who are especially sensitive to criticism may need kinder, softer words, while stubborn, aggressive children may need stricter limits.

This chapter is filled with preventive prescriptions for kids at different stages of development. Each one can be tailored to fit your child's special needs and temperament. The first one, however—Identify Tantrum Patterns—should be your initial step, no matter what your child's age. It will help you put tantrums into perspective and pinpoint key areas to work on.

℞ FOR TANTRUMS AT ANY AGE

Identify Tantrum Patterns

Before you can learn to reduce and manage temper tantrums, you need to have a clear idea of when, where, and why they occur. While it's tempting to rely on memory for these facts, if you're really serious about changing your child's behavior, you should take a more scientific approach. The best strategy is to keep a written record or chart of your child's tantrums over the course of 1 or 2 weeks (depending on how frequently tantrums occur). Though writing things down takes extra time and effort—both precious commodities in most parents' lives—it is worth it. In the long run, it'll give you a more realistic and objective view of your child's behavior. (You may even find that the tantrums aren't as bad as you thought!)

---------------------------- ✻ ----------------------------

The Birth of a Tantrum

1. Child seems unusually sullen or irritable.
2. Distraction, a hug, or other special attention doesn't seem to improve her mood.

3. She tries to do something that's beyond her ability or asks for something she's pretty sure she can't have.
4. She escalates her demand with whining and won't take no for an answer.
5. She moves on to crying, screaming, kicking, hitting, or even holding her breath: a tantrum is born.

As part of this process, it's important to enlist help from everyone who is involved in caring for your child (your spouse, babysitters, grandparents, teachers, and so on). Otherwise, the picture you get will not be complete.

How you structure your tantrum journal is not nearly as important as what you include in it. Among the most vital facts to record are:

- Who was there to witness the tantrum (you, your spouse, a babysitter, and so forth)
- When it occurred (the time, the day, and the length of the outburst)
- Where it occurred (at home, in a store, on the playground)
- What your child did before, during, and after the tantrum (Did he throw things? hurt himself? lash out at a sibling? scream and yell?)
- How you responded to the child, and how the tantrum finally ended (for example, he curled up in your lap or asked for a hug)
- Why you think your child lost control (Did age, development, or temperament play a role? Was the problem lack of sleep or hunger? Is your child getting sick?)

See below for an example of how your tantrum journal could look.

Sample Tantrum Journal

Day of week: Monday

Who:	Mom	Dad
When:	11:15–11:30 A.M.	5:00–5:30 P.M.
Where:	On the playground	At home
What:	He saw some kids eating cookies and decided he wanted one; I said no and offered fruit; he screamed and started hitting me.	It was suppertime, but he wanted to watch a video; I told him he had to wait, so he threw the video on the floor and started kicking it.
How:	I tried to offer an acceptable alternative, but he wouldn't listen, so I put him in the car; the tantrum ended when he fell asleep.	I told him he could watch the video after supper, but he kept screaming; then, when I saw him try to break the video, I got mad and told him videos were off limits for the rest of the week; then I made him go to his room; the tantrum ended when he decided he wanted to eat.
Why:	He was overtired.	Maybe he was tired after a long day of play and no nap; supper was later than usual—maybe he was hungry.

Try to be as detailed and as honest as you can in your tantrum journal. Even if you lost your temper and yelled at your child, smacked her on the bottom or gave in to what the child demanded, write it down. This is no time to pretend you're the perfect parent. As Dr. Betty Franklin points out, "You need to know exactly what is happening so you can come up with strategies and solutions that will really work."

At the end of your observation period, look closely at what you've written. You may be surprised to find that there's a certain predictability to your child's outbursts—and to your reactions. Any patterns you can identify—in terms of time, place, people, and so on—will make it that much easier for you to avoid tantrums, improve your own bad habits, and teach your child whatever she needs to learn in order to outgrow this behavior.

Once your journal is complete, set aside an afternoon or evening to sit down with your spouse and/or your child's other primary caregivers, and discuss her behavior patterns. (Even if you honestly can't find the time to keep a written record of tantrums, you should at least schedule this meeting.)

"Both parents must come to an agreement about what the problems are and map out a strategy together before specific solutions are used," says Dr. Stephen Garber, a coauthor of the book *Good Behavior*. "Also, for the sake of consistency, it will help enormously if other adults who interact regularly with your child are involved, too."

Among the questions you and your "focus group" will want to explore are the following:

Sample Tantrum-Pattern Questions

1. Is my child more likely to throw a tantrum in front of one particular person or parent? If so, what are some possible reasons why that person brings out the "worst" in my child? (For example, the child may feel less—or more—secure with that person; the adult's expectations may be out of line with the child's abilities or development; their temperaments may clash.)

2. Do tantrums tend to occur on a certain day of the week or during a certain part of the day? (The child may tend to fall apart on Fridays, after a long week of activity, or explode more frequently in the morning, rather than the afternoon.)

3. Do tantrums tend to occur in a certain place? What is it about this site (or these sites) that seems to encourage tantrums (for example, there are too many activities, toys, loud noises, things to buy)?

4. Do any of my child's stronger temperamental traits (review the worksheet in Chapter Two) play a role in when, where, how, or why my child throws tantrums? (For example, a child with a low sensory threshold may often explode when shopping for new clothes because the stiff, scratchy materials bother him.)

5. Is there any pattern to how my child acts just before a tantrum blows? during the tantrum itself? just after the tantrum is over?

6. How do I (and other caregivers) typically react to my child's tantrums? Do some responses seem to work better than others? Are certain caregivers more effective at ending tantrums than others? What can I learn about tantrum management from other adults who care for my child?

7. Are there any tantrum-response tactics that make things worse (or better) for my child (for example, trying to reason with her, hugging, spanking, and so on)?

8. How do most of my child's tantrums end, and how do different caregivers make peace when an outburst is over?

Based on your discussion and your tantrum journal, make a list of any tantrum patterns you can identify, even if there are only a few seemingly simple ones, such as "My child's most vulnerable period of the day is just before supper," or "Transitions are especially difficult for him." You'll still make a difference if you reinforce these with the anti-tantrum prescriptions that follow.

℞ FOR EARLY AND TODDLER TANTRUMS

AGE FLAG: 1 TO 3 YEARS

Avoid Tantrum Triggers

The younger your child and the less well-developed her language skills, the more you should concentrate on avoiding tantrums. This doesn't mean you should immediately give in when a tantrum occurs. If your baby or toddler wants something you don't feel she should have—whether it's another cookie, a knife she wants to play with, or a ride in the car without her carseat—you should never allow a tantrum (or the threat of a tantrum) to change your mind. But if you know your child is hungry and you're right in the middle of preparing a snack when a tantrum begins, you can calmly and quickly serve her the food without worrying that you're spoiling her or encouraging future tantrums. As Dr. Franklin points out, "With kids this young, you aren't giving in if you were going to do it anyway. You're simply avoiding an unnecessary blowout."

Avoidance doesn't mean being overprotective or trying to shield your child from stress, either. Challenges, changes, and even restrictions provide kids with important opportunities to learn and practice different skills, including how to handle frustration, anger, disappointment, and jealousy. But there is a big difference between feeling challenged and feeling overwhelmed. As Dr. Kathy Merritt observes, "A little frustration can push a child to learn and achieve; a lot, however, has the opposite effect."

It's important to understand the difference—and to try to avoid the latter. For example, if you see that your child is mildly frustrated by something (learning to use a spoon or stack blocks, for instance), you needn't jump right in to rescue him, but you should look on and be supportive, says Dr. Merritt. If his frustration starts bordering on rage, you should intervene quickly: help him out, offer an alternative, move him to another part of the room.

Similarly, if you know that a certain activity, environment, or social situation is beyond your child's capacities, avoid it—even if it's something other kids his age enjoy without a problem (like a birthday party or a trip to the state fair). In another year or two, he'll be more mature and controlled and ready to indulge. Many parents learn this strategy the hard way, through trial and error:

"When my son, Zack, was between ages 2 and 3, I refused to take him anywhere near Toys Я Us," says Carolyn Davenport. "It was just too much for him— he couldn't handle the excitement of being around all those toys. He'd always end up throwing a tantrum. I finally figured out that the best solution was to avoid that particular store until he was older and better controlled."

Others find that avoidance makes life easier not only for their child, but for them as well. "When my second child was in the tantrum stage, I learned to avoid going anywhere that might cause her conflict," says Kelly Smith. "I had two other young children around, and I knew I had to conserve my energy. Sometimes, I even had to pass up fun things. Once, a friend invited me and the kids out for a movie and ice cream, and even though I really wanted to go, I decided in the end to decline because I knew that it would be too much for my kids—and me—to handle."

Some people may think—or rudely tell you—that this approach constitutes mollycoddling. But most experts believe that it's both practical and loving, especially in the pre-preschool years. "I don't see undue frustration as the road to learning," says Dr. Merritt. "Nor is it a cop-out to help your child avoid frustrations she's not ready to handle. It's a way of giving her time to grow up—to gain the social, emotional, and experiential maturity she needs to deal with the moods and emotions that accompany tantrums."

Do's and Don'ts for Avoiding Tantrums

Don't:

• Expect your child to behave like an adult in any circumstance
• Mistake verbal ability for reasoning skills—kids can often say things that they don't really understand
• Expect a young child to have the same stamina as older children when it comes to outings at the park, the zoo, amusement parks, museums, shopping malls, and so forth (what's fun for a 5-year-old may be torture for a 2-year-old)
• Expect your child to maintain her normal levels of skill and composure if she's hungry, sick, overtired, getting used to a new babysitter or teacher, excited about a big holiday or birthday, or dealing with an unusual stress (such as death of a loved one or pet, divorce, a parent's absence, a new sibling, a new home, and so on)
• Expect your child to behave like your neighbor's, sister's, or friend's child, or to follow in the footsteps of an older sibling (every child is unique!)

Do:

• Spend time with families whose kids are about the same age as yours, so you can get a clearer sense of child development and behavior and adjust your expectations of your own child
• Temporarily hide (or resist buying) toys that are beyond your child's skill level
• Limit television and video time, and avoid programs

that are scary, violent, or designed for an older audience
* Pack plenty of snacks and toys, and plan lots of breaks when you leave the house for more than 1 hour
* Develop and (as much as possible) stick to a regular schedule of napping, eating, and playing (kids thrive on routine!)
* Watch for ways in which your temperament clashes with your child's (for example, you are extremely outgoing, so you push your child—who happens to be extremely shy—into social situations, and then get angry when she loses control)
* Get your child's other primary caregivers or teachers involved in your preventive strategy, to ensure your child hears a consistent message about how to behave

The best way to know what to avoid in order to reduce outbursts is to review your tantrum journal (or any notes taken during your tantrum discussion). Jot down the patterns you see, and then brainstorm solutions. For example, you may notice that:

• Your 16-month-old frequently has a fit when she's playing with a new puzzle she received from her aunt. She seems to love the puzzle and enjoys looking at the pieces, but when she tries to put them in their proper places, all hell breaks loose. She screams and cries, and eventually ends up flinging the puzzle and the pieces onto the floor.

   These tantrums will immediately disappear if you either put the entire puzzle away until your child's dexterity improves or keep the interesting pieces out where she can play with them and put the puzzle board away until she's ready for it. (You'll also eliminate the risk of undermining her future enjoyment of puzzles.)

· Your toddler is highly active and has a hard time sitting still for long periods of time.

Rather than subject him (and you) to long shopping trips that inevitably end in frustration and tears, you could plan to do most of your major shopping by catalog for a while, or hire a babysitter when you need to stock up on things. In 1 or 2 years, when your child is more mature and better able to sit still or amuse himself in a shopping cart, you can resume your regular shopping habits.

There are many other simple ways to make a young child's life less stressful and frustrating. Some parents, like Suzanne Koller, say their main strategy is just keeping up with the daily nap routine. "I try not to do anything new or big like food shopping close to naptime because I know my kids are especially vulnerable then," Suzanne says. "The better I can keep to a consistent sleep routine, the better they tend to do."

This isn't always easy, especially when you have more than one kid and lots of activities to taxi them to. But it is worth it to give naptime priority. Up until age 3 or 4, most kids need 12 or 13 hours of sleep each day, including 2 or so hours of naptime, according to Richard Ferber, M.D., director of the Center for Pediatric Sleep Disorders at Children's Hospital in Boston and author of *Solve Your Child's Sleep Problems.* "If they don't get sufficient daytime sleep, they get cranky, moody, overtired, and in some cases, overactive. This can lead to tantrums and other negative behaviors."

Unfortunately, around age 2, as part of their quest for independence, kids often begin resisting naps, making them a prime time for tantrums. A good way to avoid blowouts and still ensure that your child gets the rest she needs is to frame naps in a new way: tell your child it's "quiet time" or "rest period," and let her know that she doesn't have to sleep, but she does have to stay in one place and play quietly. You could even give her some special books, puzzles, or music tapes to enjoy only during this special time, or curl up on the couch or bed with her (if you need a nap, too!). If she's tired enough, the quiet activity will lull her to sleep; even if it doesn't, however, the rest will be refreshing, and will help her maintain control during the rest of the day, says Dr. Ferber.

Regularly scheduled meals and snacks are also important for young children, who are often having too much fun playing and exploring to slow down and eat. One minute they seem fine; the next minute they're as hungry as bears—and growling at you to prove it. When he was 15 months old, my younger son Teddy was especially miserable in the morning. His worst tantrums occurred when my husband and I were running around trying to get cereal in his bowl and juice in his cup. When we finally realized that the poor child was simply starving after a long night's sleep, we were able to break this bad habit instantly—by handing him a banana or cup of milk (filled the night before) while we got breakfast on the table.

Also, since hunger-induced tantrums—or, as we now fondly refer to them, "food moods"—are so com-

mon and needlessly disruptive in our household, we
never go anywhere without stuffing some crackers,
raisins, pretzels, fruit, or other healthy munchies into
the diaper bag—just in case we get delayed, we're having too much fun to leave the park, or we're stuck
in a traffic jam. (Some smart parents I know keep a
permanently stocked cooler in their car trunk.)

Here are some other simple ideas for avoiding early
and toddler tantrums:

- Childproof your house. If you have the kind of kid
  who gets into everything, make sure there isn't anything dangerous or breakable she can get into. This
  way, you won't be saying "No, don't touch that!" all
  day long, and she won't feel so frustrated when exploring.
- If your child's not athletic, don't try to force him to
  ride a tricycle just because all the other kids in the
  neighborhood do. Let him play dress-up or puzzles
  instead, and reintroduce the trike or bike in another
  year or so.
- If she's at her worst in the afternoon, plan to do
  outside errands and grocery shopping in the morning, when she's fresh and ready for adventure.
- If he's upset about a new sibling, find extra time to
  spend alone with him, and encourage him to express
  his feelings. If he asks you to throw the baby in the
  trash or bring her back to the hospital, for instance,
  don't admonish ("What a horrible thing to say! She's
  your sister and you should love her!")—acknowledge
  ("I know it's hard to have a new baby in the house,
  and it's okay if you don't like her right away. But
  she's part of our family now, so we need to keep

her"). Remember: you can't change how your child
feels, only the way he acts.

- If she has trouble sitting still, avoid situations that
  require it (like taking her to a movie theater, a nice
  restaurant, an adult concert, a long religious service)
  and find ways to break up long car rides or shopping
  trips with time for run-around play.
- If he's easily frightened, avoid violent or scary TV
  shows and books about monsters—even if he requests them or other kids his age enjoy them. What
  gives one kid the chills may give another nightmares.
  Go with your gut instinct, not your child's requests.
- If she has trouble interacting with groups of kids,
  invite only one other child to the house at a time and
  suppress the urge to throw her a huge birthday party
  until she's older.
- If he's too young to handle the excitement, keep vis-
  its to amusement parks and museums brief, and plan
  them for his most alert and active time of day.
- If she's sick, relax the household rules and routines
  until she feels better.

There are no set formulas here. Every child has his
own developmental timetable and breaking point. The
key is to watch those carefully and try to smooth your
child's way.

"I've learned, with experience, to stay very aware
of my kids' thresholds," says Elizabeth Dunn. "If I
have eight things on my agenda and notice by the time
I get to item number three that one of my girls is about
to lose control, I just turn around and go straight

home. I don't get as much done, but life is far more peaceful this way—for all of us."

Of course, avoidance isn't always possible. Sometimes, you have no choice but to forge ahead into potential tantrum territory. In such cases, your best defense is distraction. For example:

- You and your child are in a restaurant, and she suddenly gets the urge to use her fork and spoon as drumsticks.

  You feel it's too late to leave the restaurant (you've already ordered), and you're afraid that if you take the utensils away, she'll throw a loud and embarrassing fit. "Rather than make a scene, give her two straws to bang instead," advises Dr. Merritt. "Or hand her the cellophane wrapper from a pack of crackers. She can still make a little noise, but it won't disrupt everyone else's dinner."

  If all else fails, take her out to the lobby or parking lot or even to the restroom for a moment. With young children, a change of scenery is an automatic distraction.

- You're in the midst of cooking dinner when your child begins begging you to read a book.

  You can't stop cooking, but you know that if you refuse him, he'll throw a tantrum and you'll have to deal with the outburst. Rather than ignore his requests or say no, try to distract him with another play choice—stacking up plastic cups and bowls or putting spoons in and taking them out of an empty milk bottle, for instance—or ask an older sibling to read to him.

"What all this boils down to is organizing your life so that your child does not feel pushed beyond her limits," says Dr. Franklin.

This isn't always easy, of course, and it does require sacrifice. As Patricia Sutter notes, "When our twins were born, our lives turned upside down. We suddenly had to gear all our activities around their routines and schedules. During the tantrum years, we had to be especially careful about planning ahead and scheduling, so we wouldn't push them beyond their limits. Even simple things like going to church became major events that had to be scheduled and planned."

This type of juggling may be especially difficult if one of your children is "easier" than another. "My first child was the kind of baby you could take anywhere, but my second was just the opposite," says Wendy White-Hensen. "I found I had to restrict myself and my movements a lot more after he was born; it was hard not to resent that."

Unfortunately, with babies and toddlers, there aren't many other positive alternatives. Trying to "talk it out" with kids under age 2 is useless, as is expecting them to have better self-control; they simply aren't ready to respond to these strategies. Believe it or not, if all you manage to do is ease your child past the terrible twos with as few tantrums as possible, you're doing a good job.

If you find this job particularly difficult or feel avoidance and distraction aren't helping, you may need to re-examine your expectations of your child. "At some point, every parent has to move from the child they've dreamed about to the child they have," says Dr. Franklin. "Your kid may not be the great group leader or athlete you'd hoped for," she explains. "She may not be the kind of child you dreamed of, who can practice violin for 2 hours a day. She may not even be as relaxed and easy-going as you'd hoped or expected."

The sooner you can accept such disappointments, the better you'll be at understanding who your child is and what's most important and appropriate for him. "If you create a life for your child that's in harmony with his temperament and personality," says Dr. Franklin, "it will make a significant difference in his tantrum habits."

It will also make a difference in the kind of long-term relationship you develop with your child. "Whenever possible," advises Dr. Lawrence Balter, "avoid, circumscribe, or prevent tantrums, so your daily interactions with your child can be as pleasant as possible. Then, when there's an occasional tantrum (rather than daily battles), you can accept it, forget it, and move on."

℞ FOR TODDLER AND PRESCHOOL TANTRUMS

AGE FLAG: 2 TO 4 YEARS

Practice and Praise

Once you've learned to avoid certain tantrum triggers, it's important to supplement your efforts with practice and praise. While neither produces instant results, both provide young children with vital information on how they should behave. For instance, say you have a slow-to-warm-up child who tends to have tantrums when she meets new people or is thrust into new situations. "You know this child is going to have to go to

school someday," says Dr. Stella Chess, "and you
know that transition will be hard. There will be a new
building, new people, a new teacher, and new rules
and routines. Rather than force her to cope with all
those variables at once and risk a long period of intense tantrums, you can let her practice getting used
to them one at a time, in a safe environment, beforehand."

For example, you could first have her spend time
alone with an adult friend or babysitter at your house.
When she's comfortable with that, have her visit that
person's house, so she can see how the rules and routines are different there. Then, gradually increase the
amount of time she spends at the new place with the
new person, and introduce other children into the picture. "It may take more than the usual number of ex-
posures to help a shy child feel comfortable in a new
situation," says Dr. Chess, "but the more practice she
gets, the more confident she'll feel."

A good way to know what to practice with your
young child is to look again at your tantrum journal
and pinpoint some typical tantrum-producing situations. Then, in each case, try to determine what the
opposite behavior to the tantrum would be, says Dr.
Stephen Garber. "The question you need to ask," he
adds, "is not 'How can I stop the tantrums?' but 'What
do I need to teach my child, so he won't resort to tantrums?'"

For example: the opposite of throwing a tantrum
because you can't wait your turn is being able to delay
gratification and wait your turn. To help your child
learn this, you could focus on games that encourage
turn-taking (for example, handing toys back and forth,

taking turns putting blocks in a bucket, taking turns going down the slide, and so on). While you're playing, say things like "Now it's my turn! Now it's your turn!" or "I can hardly wait to get a turn!" or "It's so much fun when we take turns." Gradually, as your child's ability to wait improves, you can introduce another child into the games.

Another approach is to purposely delay your usual response time (by a few minutes) when your child is clamoring for attention while you're cooking or on the phone or talking to another adult. Bit by bit, he'll learn patience by practicing it.

As even small gains are made, be sure to praise your child for her efforts. Any time she improves a behavior, avoids throwing a tantrum, or demonstrates a better alternative for expressing her anger and frustration, notice and comment upon it—not by fawning all over her ("Oh, you are absolutely the most wonderful child ever born"), but by stating specifically what it is that pleases you: "Thank you for waiting your turn!" or "You did a great job playing quietly while I was on the phone." You can even praise the absence of a typical negative response: "You had to wait a long time, and you didn't even throw a tantrum!"

Even if your toddler doesn't understand every word you say, she'll get the message that you're pleased, and quickly catch on to the kind of behavior that wins your approval.

Be sure to make your praise specific and sincere, however. As with anything else, if you overdo it (by running around the house and clapping your hands just because your kid didn't bash his sister, for instance), it may backfire. As Dr. Williamson points out in his book *Good Kids, Bad Behavior,* "Many children love praise and will actively work to get it. But children can also get tired of praise. Moreover, if children are not used to getting praised, the loud and noisy variety will feel phony to them."

"The praise must fit the child," says Dr. Garber in agreement. "Some children like to be praised openly and lavishly; others prefer a subtle wink or thumbs-up signal. Pay attention to your child's reactions to tell whether or not you're striking the right chord. Even if he plays down your comments, but later repeats the good behavior, you'll know your approach is working."

Also, be sure you don't dilute your praise with negative comments, says James Windell. "Many parents have trouble with this, particularly those who feel very discouraged by their kids' behavior," he says. They'll say something nice like, "You did a great job sharing with your sister"—and then add a kicker—"but you should have given her the toy the first time she asked." Kids, of course, tend to remember the "but" part. "Effective praise does not include any criticism or negative remarks," says Windell. "Keep it pure and save your critical comments for some other occasion."

A good way to give verbal praise even more impact, especially with young children, is to add a pat on the head, a kiss, hug, or even a brief back rub, adds Windell. Touch is incredibly important to kids of any age.

Dr. Barbara Howard agrees and advises parents who are having significant problems with their child's behavior to go even further. "Whenever you notice your child acting appropriately—or not acting inappropriately—take a green (washable) marker and put a mark on the back of his hand as you deliver the verbal praise," she says. "This will bring eye contact and touching into the picture, both of which have a powerful effect on children."

When you give the green marks is not as important as how many you give, she adds. For example, you can designate anything from 10 minutes to a whole day as a "green-dot period," or use the marker only during a specific tantrum-producing situation (such as during a shopping trip). Either way, you should aim for giving a total of six to 10 dots per hour. "Fewer dots means you're not paying enough attention to your child's behavior or rewarding small enough behaviors," says Dr. Howard. "What you really want to do," she adds, "is catch your child being good."

At the end of your designated green-dot period, you can give your child a small reward (stickers, a balloon, a cookie, a trip to the park) for getting a predetermined number of marks. (For example, "If you get six green dots for good behavior while we're in the mall, you can pick out two new stickers for your album; if you get 10 dots, you can choose four new stickers!")

If necessary, after about three days of using only green marks, you can add in red dots for undesirable behavior, and then give a reward only if the green dots exceed the red dots. But very often, kids are so motivated to get those green dots, you don't even need the red marker, Dr. Howard says.

Systematic praise coupled with touch can be especially effective in reducing tantrums that have no apparent source or pattern. Often, if outbursts happen anytime, anywhere, with little warning, the underlying problem is simply lack of self-control. Giving a green dot and complementing your child when she demon- strates any degree of control helps her understand the importance and value of this difficult skill. (For exam- ple, "You did a great job behaving in that store"; "Thank you so much for being patient while I talked to the lady at the bank"; "I was so pleased that you didn't lose your temper when your friend grabbed your toys.")

Praising also gives you a chance to balance any negative interactions you've had over tantrums with some positive attention. As Dr. George Cohen points out, "If the only time a child gets attention is when she's throwing a tantrum, the outbursts will continue. Parents must make time to interact positively with their children when no tantrums are going on. That way, the child can see the parent as someone who's loving, caring and supportive—rather than as the enemy."

But, again, don't overdo it. As Dr. Garber notes, "Once a new behavior is well established, you needn't continue praising it constantly. You could notice it every fifth or tenth time it happens. But never stop praising completely."

AGE FLAG: 2 TO 4 YEARS

Label Emotions

As your child matures and his verbal skills grow, you should add another valuable element to the prevention process: labeling. What this basically entails is telling your young child what he's feeling, so his emotions won't seem so random and powerful. For example:

- If your child is having trouble getting an oval shape to fit into his shape sorter and he's giving off warning signs that a tantrum's about to blow, stop the game, get on the floor, and say to him, "It looks like you're frustrated. Let me help" or "This game is too frustrating. Let's find another."
- If she's at a birthday party and you can see that all the noise and excitement are making her wild, take her aside and say, "You seem a little overwhelmed by all this noise and excitement. Let's go outside for a minute and take a break; then we can come back."
- If he's really angry because you won't give him a cookie before dinner, tell him: "You look really angry about not getting a cookie before supper. I know it's hard to wait for a treat, and you're feeling impatient, but in this house, we eat our dinner before dessert."

There are no special tricks here: all you need do is briefly describe to your child what is happening. If you want to go even further, you can make a game of it. One technique that Dr. Garber uses involves making a "feeling" tree. First, you and your child draw a big picture of a tree. Then, you identify different feelings (mad, sad, glad, and so on) and draw a face to represent each one. Then, you place each face on the tree, with a word describing it underneath, and cut out some pictures from magazines to illustrate the different feelings. Paste those on the tree, too. "Once the tree is finished, you can use it as a prompt to help the child label his feelings," says Dr. Garber.

The more your child talks about feelings and hears you describe them, the better he'll get at identifying them himself; this will later help him in controlling his emotions. But don't just concentrate on the four biggies—mad, sad, glad, and scared—warns Dr. Williamson. Try to also label behavior that's less clear-cut. "Very often, kids are reacting to what I call the 'feeling that has no name'—that excited, wound-up, restless, fidgety stuff," he says. "When you see it happening, describe it, and give it a name. For example, say, 'When I see you hopping around like that and talking in that loud voice, it tells me you're feeling wound up and you need to take a break.' After hearing your description 300 or 400 times, your child will be able to name it himself. Then he'll be ready to take steps to control it, too."

Another effective way to help your child identify and understand emotions is to read her books about other kids with similar feelings, says Karen Buchanan of Project Enlightenment. (For a list of suggested books, see page 111.) "Reading together is a wonderful way for parents to help young children learn and talk about their feelings. It also helps send the message that it's okay to be angry and frustrated, and that there are healthy ways to express and control these emotions."

Books to Share with Your Child

Here is a sampling of the many books on tantrums, anger, and other emotions that you can share with your child. Check your local library for more listings.

Picture Books (Ages 2 to 5)

Angry Arthur, by Hiawyn Oram; illustrated by Satoshi Kitamura (Dutton)

Feelings, by Aliki (Greenwillow)

Pookins Gets Her Way, by Helen Lester; illustrated by Lynn Munsinger (Houghton Mifflin)

Poopy the Panda, by Dick Gackenbach (Clarion)

Preschool and Early Reader Books (Ages 3 to 6)

Alexander and the Terrible, Horrible, No Good, Very Bad Day, by Judith Viorst; illustrated by Ray Crutz (Atheneum)

Dinah's Mad, Bad Wishes, by Barbara M. Josse; illustrated by Emily Arnold McCully (HarperCollins)

Don't Forget to Come Back, by Robie H. Harris; illustrated by Tony DeLuna (Alfred A. Knopf)

Don't Throw Another One, by Beverly Lou Keller; illustrated by Jacqueline Chwast (Coward, McCann & Geoghegan)

Even If I Did Something Awful, by Nancy Kincade (Atheneum)

How Do I Feel? and *I Was So Mad,* by Norma Simon; illustrated by Joe Laskar (Albert Whitman)

I Was So Mad by Mercer Mayer, Golden Press

Let's Talk about Throwing Tantrums, by Joy Wilt Berry; illustrated by John Costanza (Children's Press)

No One is Perfect, by Karen Erickson; illustrated by Maureen Roffey (Viking)

The Tantrum, by Kathryn Lasky; illustrated by Bobette McCarthy (Macmillan)

The Temper Tantrum Book, by Edna Mitchell Preston; illustrated by Rainey Bennett (Scholastic Inc.)

When Emily Woke Up Angry, by Riana Duncan (Barron's Educational Series)

———————————— ✳ ————————————

Another good tool, Buchanan says, is role playing. "I strongly encourage parents to use puppets, dolls, and even superhero toys to help their kids open up about feelings and talk about alternative reactions," she says. For example, if you and your child are playing with some superhero figures, you could work in a conversation like this:

> I have Trini, and she looks really mad because she can't find her power crystal. Uh-oh, she's starting to throw things around and yell about it. Look at how she's acting. Now the other superheroes are afraid of her because she looks so mad. What should she do instead to get them to help her look for it?

Try to get your child involved in brain-storming solutions, and encourage him to talk about things that make him (or his superhero) really mad or frustrated. But keep in mind that you are playing with your child. You don't want to stir up angry feelings or aggressive behavior by letting the game become violent. Nor should you use this time to lecture, reprimand or remind your child of his past sins (as in "You were acting just like Trini yesterday, weren't you?" or "Nobody's going to want to be your friend, either, if you keep acting like her"). Instead, concentrate on sharing ideas and labeling emotions in an easy, relaxed, pressure-free manner ("She looks pretty angry to me. What do you think? What would your guy do?") If your child seems too uncomfortable or doesn't feel like going along with the game, end it. But don't stop looking for ways to label. As Dr. Garber points out, "Identifying feelings is a skill that always needs refining, so look for opportunities whenever you can."

℞ FOR PRESCHOOL TANTRUMS

AGE FLAG: 3 TO 4 YEARS

Encourage Control

The better your child gets at labeling and expressing her emotions, the more you should focus on encouraging self-control. While avoidance of undue frustration is still useful—especially when it comes to scheduling your child's day and signing her up for other activities—it's not as practical in the preschool years. As your child ventures forth to school, play groups, sports teams, and other social events, your control over what she's exposed to will naturally dwindle.

This is as it should be. By age 3 or 4, most kids are ready to take on increasing challenges from the world at large. They have a better understanding of their emotions, their body control has improved, and their language skills are developing rapidly. In fact, by now, if gently reminded, most kids are able to use their words rather than their bodies when expressing emotions. (If a child is suffering from a language delay, however, this may be more difficult, and your expectations should be different. Consult your pediatrician or a speech-language pathologist if pronunciation or communication problems persist after age 3.)

Are You Listening?

If you want your child to learn to use words—rather than feet or fists—when expressing anger and frustration, you must be prepared to listen. That means:

* Stopping whatever it is you're doing and looking directly at your child when she has a pressing complaint
* Repeating back what you've heard without judgment, even if you don't agree or the complaint makes you angry ("It sounds like you are really angry because I cut the crusts off your sandwich")
* Resisting the urge to:
  * "Correct" your child's feelings ("Oh, you don't really mean that"; "That's a terrible thing to say")
  * Minimize them ("There's nothing to be upset about"; "You're making a big deal out of nothing")
  * Teach a lesson ("See, I told you that would happen")
* Setting limits on her use of abusive words and violent behavior ("I know you're angry, but in this house we don't call names"; "I can see why you're frustrated, but it's not okay to break things or hurt your brother")
* Showing the child you've heard her, even if you can't change what happened ("I'm really sorry you feel that way, but I can't glue crusts back onto a sandwich; I'll make myself a special note, so I'll remember not to cut them off again tomorrow")

One way to give your child a sense of control is to demystify tantrums—or make them seem less scary and powerful—by using them in games. "My favorite technique is to pick a time when the child is happy and throw a mock tantrum in her presence," says Marilyn Segal, Ph.D., developmental psychologist and dean of the Family and School Center at Nova Southeastern University, in Fort Lauderdale, Florida. "For instance, you might say, 'Oh, I'm so angry. I thought I left my shoes right here in the hallway, but now I can't find them. That's it, I'm going to have a tantrum. Let's see, first I've got to make some funny noises—argh, rarh, blah. Now, I'd better stamp my feet. What else should I do? Wave my arms? Okay, how's this? Oh, yeah, I forgot to make a mad face . . .'. If you can get the child involved in describing how to behave during a tantrum, and show her how silly you look having one, it helps her see that tantrums are something harmless that she really can control."

"Once the game is over, you can ask your child, 'What do you think I could have done instead of having a tantrum?'" says Dr. Segal. "It'll help her think of alternative behaviors without making her feel like she's the one who did something wrong."

Another fun way to help your child learn she has control over tantrums is to time them, says Dr. Segal. "Rather than telling the child outright that the tantrums have to stop, say, 'Let's see. The last time you had a tantrum it lasted for 9 minutes. The next time you have one, I'll put the timer on for 7 minutes, and we'll see if you can stop your tantrum before the buzzer goes off.' Once temper tantrums become something you can talk about and manipulate," adds Dr.

Segal, "you'll be amazed at how quickly they go away."

Foreshadowing is another useful technique for helping preschool-age kids feel they have more control
over how they act. Children this young often throw
tantrums when they don't know what's going to happen to them or can't understand what the adults
around them want or expect. Remember: what you
may see as a routine visit to the dentist, the mall,
or even a grandparent's house, your child may view
as a new and potentially dangerous adventure. You
will allay many of his fears just by giving a brief
explanation of what's going to happen, how you want
him to behave, and what to do if he begins to feel
overwhelmed.

While you don't want to be too long-winded, you
should try to cover the following six points when preparing your child for a new or potentially tantrum-
producing situation:

1. Acknowledge how your child feels. ("I know that
   you have a hard time sitting still in the cart when
   we go to the store because it gets boring, and you
   see lots of things there you want to buy . . .")
2. Explain why it's important for him to behave.
   (". . .but I really need to pick up a few things for
   supper.")
3. Describe how you expect him to behave. ("I need
   you to sit quietly in the cart and not whine and cry
   for things we don't need to buy today.")
4. Suggest coping strategies. ("Why don't we bring
   your new book with us, so you can read it if you
   get bored? Is there anything else you'd like to bring
   to play with?")

5. Offer an incentive for good behavior. ("If you can sit quietly and play with your toys while I shop, I'll finish faster and we can spend some extra time at the playground before dinner.")
6. State the consequences for having a tantrum. ("If you throw a tantrum or whine and cry for things I can't buy, I'll have to stand still and wait for you to finish; I won't talk to you until you're calm, and then I'll finish the shopping, and we'll come straight home—with no time for the playground.")

Be sure to speak in a matter-of-fact tone of voice, and avoid saying anything that might make your child feel ashamed or guilty for past behavior (such as "You're always such a whiner when we go into stores" or "You're so greedy, you want everything"). And no matter what your child's past history, act like you have confidence in her ability to succeed this time around. (If controlling your voice and words is difficult, pretend you're talking to a new employer or a neighbor—someone you'd never dream of being rude to—rather than your tantrum-prone child.)

If your child ends up throwing a tantrum anyway, don't launch into a lecture or call names (as in "I thought we agreed that you'd behave" or "There you go acting like a baby again. You can just forget about the park or any other fun thing now"). Instead, follow through on your plan without discussion, and repeat this process the next time a similar situation is about to occur. (For more on this, see "Set Limits," on page 121.)

Another good time to foreshadow is right before a transition. For example, if you need to leave the park by noon, give your child a 10-minute warning ("I know you're having fun, but we have to leave in 10 more minutes to get home for lunch. Is there one more thing you'd like to play on?"); then a 5-minute warning ("Five more minutes, and then it's time to go"); and, if necessary, a 1-minute warning ("One more minute"). That way, he won't feel helpless or throw a tantrum because you're whisking him away in the middle of play.

If it's almost time to leave for the babysitter's but your child is engrossed in coloring, you could strengthen your warning by setting a timer: "You can color for 5 more minutes, and then we have to go to Samantha's. I'll put on the timer so you'll know we have to go when the bell rings"). As Dr. Merritt points out, "This will help you avoid last-minute arguments and the inevitable pleas for 'one more minute!'" If your child protests, you can always throw up your hands and say, innocently, "The timer went off. Time to go." Kids find it far less gratifying to argue with a kitchen gadget than with a parent.

Yet another effective technique for fostering self-control is giving choices whenever possible, says Dr. Howard. This does not include emotionally charged choices such as "Do you want to spend the weekend with me or your father?" (in the case of a divorce). It's not fair to ask a child to make a decision like that.

Nor should you offer open-ended choices. If you have a child who routinely throws tantrums in the morning because "you didn't give me the right cereal," a question such as "What do you want to eat this morning?" will inevitably lead to disaster. Your child will name the most sugary or obscure brand he can think of, and when you tell him you don't have that cereal in the house, he'll take it as proof of his right to explode.

A better approach is to offer two specific and realistic choices: "Which would you like to eat today, Cheerios or Kix?" Make sure either choice is acceptable to you, and then let your child make the weighty decision. If he just can't decide, and you're in a hurry to get out of the house, give him a third choice: "If you can't decide, I'll have to decide for you, and I'll pick Kix."

Once a choice is made, praise your child for being so decisive (for example, "Great choice"). Use this strategy over and over again, in as many situations you can. As Dr. Crockenberg points out, "The best way to gain compliance and avoid defiance in a young child is to offer clear directives and some kind of autonomy sharing (choices)."

℞ FOR PRESCHOOL AND BIG-KID TANTRUMS

AGE FLAG: 3 TO 6 YEARS

Teach Relaxation

Another way to help your child improve her self-control is by training her to relax her body when she begins to feel stressed. "The relaxation response is not automatic," notes Dr. Garber. "Kids—as well as adults—must learn it and practice it."

A good way to begin is to teach your child (and yourself!) the most relaxing way to breathe: from the diaphragm, rather than the chest. Dr. Garber's approach (detailed in his book *Monsters Under the Bed and Other Childhood Fears*) goes like this:

1. Tell your child you're going to teach him something called "deep belly breathing," which he can use to relax when he's feeling frustrated or overwhelmed.
2. Have him lie flat on his back, with his arms by his sides and his legs straight.
3. Tell him to imagine that his stomach is a balloon, and ask him to try filling it up with air as he inhales.
4. Tell him not to breathe from the chest, push his stomach out, or arch his back as he breathes.
5. Place a book on his stomach, so he can better visualize the correct breathing motion.
6. Ask him to practice deep belly breathing with you for a few minutes every day, until he gets the hang of it.
7. Once he's learned to breathe from his belly, have him slow his breathing down by counting out loud to three as he inhales, and then to five as he exhales.
8. Next, teach him to slowly say the word *relax* when he exhales.

It may take a while for your child to catch on and learn to use deep belly breathing when he's on the edge of losing control. But you can help him associate the two by labeling pre-tantrum behavior and suggesting that he try deep belly breathing when you see it ("You look like you're feeling overwhelmed. Why don't you take a few deep belly breaths and then try to tell me what's wrong"). Another good way to encourage belly breathing is to do it yourself. If your child sees you using this technique to cool down, it will seem even more natural. Eventually—after many, many repetitions—your patience and his practice will pay off, and he'll have a relaxation tool he can use for the rest of his life.

You should also encourage your child to discover other activities that help her relax—sports, music, drawing, reading, riding her bike, and so forth—and make sure there's plenty of time for her to indulge in at least one every day.

℞ FOR BIG-KID TANTRUMS

AGE FLAG: 4 TO 6 YEARS

Set Limits

For older children who have intense temper outbursts or routinely use tantrums to manipulate others, a direct discussion of acceptable and unacceptable behavior is in order—and it should include significant limit setting. The goal, at this point, is to help your child understand that while her emotions and desires are normal, her behavior needs to improve, and only she can improve it.

Some Healthy Alternatives for Handling Anger

* Saying "I'm angry!" and telling an adult why (without calling names, blaming, or hurting the other person's feelings)
* Growling like a lion

- Making ugly faces in the mirror
- Kicking a ball around outside
- Going outside and yelling at the sky
- Hitting a pillow, stuffed animal, punching bag, or other inanimate object that can't be broken or hurt
- Drawing a picture about how you feel—and then ripping it up
- Ripping up old newspapers, magazines, or junk mail set aside in a special "ANGER" box
- Going for a bike ride or stomping around outdoors
- Writing about angry feelings in a special notebook

There is no one right way to have a tantrum discussion, but there are some guidelines that will help you keep the conversation positive:

1. Pick a time when things are calm (your child hasn't just had a tantrum, and you're not feeling angry) to talk about tantrums. Make sure the TV is off and the answering machine is on.

2. In a gentle (not angry) tone of voice, tell your child that you've noticed she's having a hard time controlling her temper, and that it's your job to help her find better ways to express her emotions. Choose words that won't make her feel guilty, ashamed, or defensive, but be clear that tantrums are no longer going to work in your household. You might even say something like "I know that in the past, I've sometimes gotten mad at you or given in when you've had an outburst, but from now on I'm not going to do that. I can't let tan-

trums work anymore because you're too old to be throwing them."

3. Be as simple and direct as possible. If you talk too much, or go into long-winded explanations, she'll get confused and tune you out.

4. Make it clear that there's nothing wrong or abnormal about feeling angry or frustrated, but that there are better ways to express those feelings. You might say, "Everyone gets angry and frustrated now and then. Some kids your age like to punch their pillow or rip up papers or talk to an adult when they're mad. I like to take a deep breath and walk around outside. Can you think of anything you could do instead of throwing a tantrum that might make you feel better when you're angry?" Or, if manipulative tantrums are the main problem, you may want to help your child improve her negotiation skills: "You know I'm not going to give in to tantrums anymore. Let's talk about some better ways you can ask for things you want." Help her find the words to be persuasive and polite.

5. Encourage your child to come up with alternative behaviors by role-playing with him. Bring up his most recent tantrum and talk about how he was feeling, then ask him how he could have handled the situation differently. Based on his response, make a suggestion for the next time he feels the same way. For example, you might say, "It sounds like last time you were really angry because I was talking for a long time on the phone when you wanted to play. I'm sorry you felt that way, but

sometimes parents need to make plans over the phone. Maybe next time, instead of screaming and hitting me, you could color a picture about how you're feeling and then, when you can't wait any longer, hold it up for me to see. Then, if I can break away, I will; if I can't, I'll stop talking to let you know how much longer I'll be."

6. If your child doesn't like your idea or has another one of his own, listen and be supportive. Encourage him to develop a plan of action he'll feel comfortable following the next time he's frustrated. Then say, "That sounds like a great idea. Why don't we practice it right now. You pretend you're about to have a tantrum, and then go do (whatever his plan is). How did it feel? Great. Let's try that out the next time you feel like you're going to have a tantrum."

7. Let your child know you're serious by also setting limits on his tantrum behavior: "I really want to help you learn to control your temper, so if your plan doesn't work, I'll have to put 'Plan B' into action."

"Plan B" should not be a punishment, but some type of break that helps your child pull himself together. You may even want to give it a special name, such as "cool-down" time. Then, when your child explodes, you can send him to his room, or to a special cool-down chair, and ask him to stay put until he's calm enough to speak in a normal voice (for more on this, see Chapter Five). Explain the plan clearly to your child. You could even say, "Remember, if I send you out to the porch during a tantrum, it's not because I want to punish you, but because you need some privacy so you can calm down."

If a tantrum turns aggressive—your child starts hitting people or breaking things—a stronger response is in order. Instead of cool-down, call "time-out." Send your child to a predetermined spot for a specific amount of time (usually 1 minute per year of the child's age). Let her know this is more than a break—it's a consequence for misbehavior. You might say, "You're in time-out for 3 minutes for hitting." Then set a timer. When it goes off, check on the child. If she's still out of control, reset the timer.

With older kids—especially hard-core or chronic tantrum-throwers—you may want to put privileges or objects into time-out. For instance, if your child frequently has a fit because he wants to watch two videos, even though he knows the family rule is one a day, you can say, "The family rule is one video a day. You can choose the video you want, but if you throw a tantrum when it's over, I'll put both of them in time-out, and there will be no video tomorrow." Similarly, if she frequently explodes when it's time to go to bed, you can put the privilege of reading a book with you in time-out. Whatever you choose, however, make sure the consequence for throwing a tantrum is fair and logical—not overly punitive.

8. When setting limits on tantrum behavior, you need to be clear and direct. Be sure you spell out exactly:

- What type of behavior constitutes a tantrum (such as hitting or throwing things when he's frustrated, whining when he doesn't get his way, screaming and stomping around the house when he's mad)
- Why you want it to stop (because she's old enough to use more grown-up ways to express her emotions; it disrupts the household and gets everyone else wound up, and so on)
- At what point you will try to stop it (for example, as soon as you hear him scream or see him hitting someone; as soon as you notice him getting whiny)
- How you will try to stop it (by putting the child in cool-down time or just ignoring him until he calms down)
- What will happen when the tantrum ends (for example, you'll listen to his complaint or try to help him out, but you won't give in)

9. Ask your child if he has any questions; then have him repeat back to you what the coping plan and consequences are, to make sure he understands them.

10. Most important, follow through exactly as you promised when any new tantrums occur. Do not let your child convince you to "give him another chance" or change your strategy, and do not escalate your consequence just because your child resists you (for example, "All right. If you aren't going into cool-down time, you can forget about watching your video this afternoon"). Even if your plan is not as successful as you'd hoped, it's

important to stick with it, so your child will know you mean business. You can always change it later, when things are calm again. (For tips on what to do if your child refuses to go into cool-down or time-out, see Chapter Five).

Following through on consequences may be exhausting, but it's vital. If you waver or suddenly change your plan or increase your punishment, your child will learn three things you'll wish he hadn't:

1. You're not serious about the limits you set.
2. You can't control your own behavior.
3. Tantrums do work.

None of the above will reduce tantrums. Consistency, however, will. As James Windell notes, "With older kids especially, the certainty of a consequence is far more likely to teach a lesson than the severity of the consequence. Kids won't change a behavior unless they're sure you're serious about what you say."

✾ FIVE

A Ton of Cure

No matter how sound your prevention strategy, it won't completely eliminate tantrums—especially if your child has a "difficult" temperament. There will still be unforeseen and unavoidable frustrations that cause your child to melt down or explode, and there will still be days when your child is feeling too sick or tired to cope with even the slightest amount of stress.

In fact, until your kid outgrows tantrums (with prevention and patience, that day will come!), the best you can hope for is not an end to all outbursts but a way to manage them, so they don't harm either your child or your relationship.

In other words, you still need to know how to deal with a loud, angry, out-of-control kid. And you'll need this skill more than ever once you get serious about prevention. As soon as your child realizes that you're out to terminate tantrums, they'll probably intensify for a while: she won't want to give up her favorite coping mechanism, so she'll first try to see how serious you are by testing you; then when she realizes you're committed to your plan, she'll fight to the bitter end to change your mind.

"Your child is going to feel the way most of us do when we don't get the candy we paid for from a vending machine," says Dr. Stephen Garber. "He'll shake, and kick, and pound before he accepts the fact that the usual pay-off isn't going to come."

Your best defense is being prepared. Just knowing you have a straightforward plan for reacting to tantrums can give you the confidence to face your child's outbursts with a clear head and calm demeanor. As James Windell notes, "Parents are most likely to overreact or react inappropriately when they feel like they don't know what to do."

Tempting Tactics That Just Don't Work

When your child's temper flares, you may be tempted to try one of the following. Resist: These are known tantrum triggers.

Tactic	Likely Result
Arguing	Further infuriates child, who is beyond reason during a tantrum
Demanding that the tantrum end	Increases child's frustration and escalates tantrum behavior

Tactic	Likely Result
Giving in	Teaches child to use temper tantrums to manipulate others
Lecturing	Increases frustration and rage; falls on deaf ears anyway
Pleading	Gives child too much power, and may scare and further enrage him
Punishing	Helps child see you as the enemy, rather than as her primary support
Shaming	Heightens child's frustration and lowers self-esteem
Yelling	Intensifies everyone's emotions and provides a poor model of self-control

---------------------------- ✳ ----------------------------

Unfortunately, there is no one trick that will tame all tempers. Every child and every tantrum situation is different; what works for one kid or one incident may not work for another. Parents need to be flexible and creative. "If you only have one solution, you're much more likely to fail," says Dr. Peter Williamson. "Your child will search and search until she sees a weak spot in your plan, and then she'll rip right through it."

"That's how it is with Grace," says Carol Spelman. "Just when I've figured out the best way to handle something Grace does, she figures me out—and jumps one step ahead."

To avoid this, you need a master plan with plenty of options. That way, if one approach doesn't work, you can shift your response quickly and efficiently, without losing ground. You pretty much want to be on automatic pilot when a tantrum occurs (unless you're particularly good at thinking creatively when someone is screaming in your face or kicking your shins), so it pays to plan ahead.

In My Experience . . .

The worst way to handle a tantrum . . . "is to try to reason with my child. It only upsets her more. Since I'm usually the one who provoked the tantrum (by saying no to something), the last thing she wants from me is a diatribe on rules and reasons. Consoling attempts also seem to intensify tantrums."

What works best for me . . . "is telling my child that I understand why she is angry, that I love her, and that I'll be here for her when she feels better. Then I just sit nearby and let her work it out. I *try* to be an impartial observer."

—Carol Spelman
mother of Grace, age 2

The following response plan—which you can adopt and adapt for different situations—will help. It starts with some basic, tried-and-true tactics (especially useful with younger children), and then takes you beyond, just in case a tantrum escalates. Each time an outburst occurs, try to start with Level 1 and work your way up; always end with Level 5. This will enable you to present a consistent (but flexible) response to your child; it will also help you see when progress is being made (when you only have to go to Level 3, instead of the usual Level 4, for instance).

You should also get in the habit of timing your child's tantrums and jotting down their length, says Dr. Garber. "This is purely to help you persist, in case you begin to feel like you're getting nowhere," he explains. If you keep a written record, you'll eventually see, in black and white, that your child has shaved off 5 minutes from his average tantrum time or is throwing fewer tantrums. Then you'll know your plan is working. It may not be working as quickly or as completely as you'd hoped, but it is working, and you should stay with it.

"Very often, parents get discouraged when they try out a new discipline technique and it 'doesn't work' with their child," adds Dr. Williamson. "But usually it's not the technique or the child that's the problem, it's the parent's expectations." Instant results are very rare in the world of child rearing. It often takes hundreds of repetitions to convince a kid—especially a strong-willed one—to change or improve a behavior. "Most children will resist you and test you first," says Dr. Williamson. "That's normal and healthy; it's their job to test and learn. But it's your job as a parent to be firm, consistent, and patient."

If you use the prevention prescriptions outlined in Chapter Four and follow the reaction techniques described in this chapter, you cannot fail. You may not obliterate tantrums, but you will reduce them, and you'll manage those that happen in a healthy way—

without losing your own temper, lashing out at your child, or resorting to harsh punishment. This may not feel like success to you, but in the world of temper tantrums, it's the pinnacle.

You won't be able to appreciate the effects of healthy tantrum management for many more years, of course. But someday, when your tantrum-prone baby, toddler, or preschooler has grown into a well-adjusted, reasonably controlled, self-confident kid, you'll know your strategy worked.

Until then, be patient, and learn to lean on the following techniques when tantrums take over and tempers flare.

How to Respond to a Temper Tantrum

Level 1: Ensure Safety

As soon as a tantrum begins, quickly assess your child's behavior for safety: Is he at risk of hurting himself? another person? surrounding property? "Most tantrums—even those involving breath-holding or head-banging—are not as dangerous as they look," says Dr. Chess. "Kids may want attention, but they rarely want to hurt themselves." (For more on breath-holding and head-banging, see pages 142 and 143.)

Still, if you have any doubts about possible injury, you should take action. If your child emerges from a tantrum with a bump on her head or a scratch on her leg, it may confirm her greatest fear: that her feelings are so powerful and dangerous, no one can protect her. This, of course, will only fuel more tantrums.

To avoid injuries, here are your basic options.

℞ FOR EARLY AND TODDLER TANTRUMS

AGE FLAG: 1 TO 3 YEARS

Removal

If your child starts throwing a tantrum in the middle of a busy street, on a staircase or in some other potentially dangerous area, pick him up immediately and carry him to a safer place. You needn't say a word as you do this, but if you feel must explain, make it simple: "I need to move you to a safer place." This may not make your child happier, but it should provide some reassurance.

"The biggest fear most kids have when they're in the midst of a tantrum is, 'Can anyone handle me?'," notes Karen Buchanan of Project Enlightenment. "If you use the word *safe* in whatever you say, it will help the child feel like someone out there is in control."

Removal is also recommended when your child is throwing a tantrum in a restaurant, theater, place of worship, or other public area where excessive noise is not welcome. This is more good manners than anything else, but it may also help you avoid giving in to your child out of sheer embarrassment.

Holding

If your child isn't in danger, but property or other people are, hold her. Pick her up, sit her in your lap on a soft couch or chair or on the floor, and wrap your arms firmly but gently around hers; if necessary, wrap your legs around hers, too, to prevent kicking.

If she's too large to sit on your lap or too strong to

hold in this position, try lying her on the floor, stomach down, and gently holding her arms at the wrists or her legs at the ankles. If she squirms and cries "You're hurting me!", reassure her that you don't want to do that. Say something like "I love you and I want to help you regain control. But I can't let you hurt yourself or break things. I will let you go as soon as you calm down."

In My Experience . . .

The worst way to handle a tantrum . . . "is to give in to the child's request or demand. I would be setting myself up for many, many more tantrums if I allowed my son to change my mind (or whatever decision he was unhappy about) by having a tantrum. A tantrum must not be used as a tool to get what he wants."

What works best for me . . . "is being very patient, and very, very calm during the tantrum. I tell my child that I love him and give him alternative choices (such as 'We can't have a friend over right now, but I'll play a game or read a book with you'). Then I ask him to let me know when he decides between the choices, and I very calmly go about my business (doing housework or whatever) while very discreetly watching him."

—Trudy Eaton
mother of Sara, age 10,
and Ross, age 5

While holding worsens tantrums in some kids (and shouldn't be enforced with them), many children—even those who protest it—find physical contact comforting when they're feeling out of control, says Dr. Kathy Merritt (see also "Hugging," under "Level 4: Contain the Chaos"). But the contact must be loving, not angry. If you can't keep your own emotions in check, you should avoid any physical contact during a tantrum.

If holding seems to be working, embrace your child firmly until you feel the anger and frustration drain from her body. You may want to repeat a soothing phrase, such as "It's okay," or "You're going to be fine," but don't attempt to talk your child out of his mood or justify what's happening. The less said during a tantrum, the better. Eventually, your child will run out of steam and snuggle into your arms. Then you can proceed to Level 5.

If holding is not working—either because your child is too strong or violent, or you are too angry—put him in his crib, high chair, stroller, or play pen and proceed to Level 2.

℞ FOR PRESCHOOL AND BIG-KID TANTRUMS

AGE FLAG: 3 TO 6 YEARS

Time-out

If an older child is hitting, biting or hurting someone, or is thrashing about within striking distance of glasses, bottles, figurines, or other breakable objects, intervene. Protect the person who is being hurt by picking your child up or pulling her away, and saying firmly: "Time-out for hurting. Three minutes (or longer, depending on the child's age)."

If you are the person being scratched or hurt, extricate yourself and walk away. Tell your child she is in time-out for aggression, and send her to the predetermined time-out spot (as discussed in Chapter Four). As one expert notes, "Your child should never be allowed to hit or hurt you. It would be too damaging to her sense of her relationship with you."

In My Experience . . .

The worst way to handle a tantrum . . . "is to yell at your child or say things like 'Go on, keep on crying. Keep it up.' Once, out of frustration, my husband said this to our 17-month-old son, and it seemed to prolong and intensify the tantrum. We have never done it since!"

What works best for me . . . "is to walk away and give the child time to cry and kick, without saying anything. Then, after a few minutes, I go and hug the child, and talk softly, telling her I love her. That usually calms her down."

—Suzanne Koller
mother of Christopher, age 5,
and Katherine, age 2

If the child follows you around and won't stop hitting or kicking, calmly put her in her room, close the door, and firmly say, "No hitting allowed. You can come out of time-out when you're finished hitting," or "In this house, we hit pillows when we're angry, not people."

If this also fails—because your child keeps coming out of the room to hunt you down and continue the tantrum in your presence—you may need to lock yourself in another room and tell your child firmly, "You are not allowed to hurt me." This will not only protect you and reinforce your point, it will help you resist the urge to hit back.

If property is in danger, remove it from your child's reach or lead your child to a kid-proofed area, while saying something like "It's okay to be angry, but it's not okay to break things." Make sure any verbal interaction you have with your child is brief, firm, calm, and direct, however. This is not the time to lecture your child on the morality of violence or the need to respect other people's property. Your only goal is to make sure everyone and everything is safe.

LEVEL 2: CALM DOWN

Once you've ensured safety, let your child kick and scream on her own for a while, so you can gather your wits. In order to react effectively to a temper tantrum, you must be calm, cool, and collected—at least to all outward appearances. Inside, you may be boiling over with rage and resentment, but you can't let your kid know this. "If you sink to the level of your child and have an adult version of a tantrum, you forfeit your chance to be an effective role model and credible teacher," says Dr. Stanley Turecki. "Plus, you risk saying or doing things you don't really mean."

In addition, you'll likely increase your child's anxiety. "When a kid is out of control, he needs to feel that there's an adult around who can save him," says

Dr. George Cohen. "He's depending on you to be the calm one, his savior."

✳

In My Experience . . .

The worst way to handle a tantrum . . . "is to act out of control or to get mad at the child. I realized with my second child that part of her feels really out of control during a tantrum, and that the calmer I am, the shorter the tantrums last."

What works best for me . . . "is remaining calm, getting the child home if we're in public, and comforting her when the tantrum is over."

—Kelly Smith
mother of James, age 9,
Kathy, age 8,
and Lillith, age 5

✳

As long as your child is safe, there's no danger in taking a few minutes to get a grip on your own emotions. In fact, this is so crucial, you should force yourself to do it even if you're in the middle of a crowded department store. The momentary embarrassment this may cause is far less serious than what you might do or say if you lose control.

To help yourself relax, you may want to:

• Close your eyes and take a few slow, deep breaths (breathing from your diaphragm, not your chest); say a soothing word, like *relax*, as you exhale

- Count to 100—and then back again

- Repeat to yourself some sort of soothing mantra, such as:

  "This is just a phase, it soon will pass."

  "I can't control my child, but I can control myself."

  "I do not know anybody in this store; I will never see any of these people again."

  "My child is not out to get me; he is acting his age."

  "This is normal behavior. I need to stay calm, so I can help."

  "I'm the adult. I need to act like one."

  "Stay calm. Stay calm. Stay calm."

- Walk away from your child until you cool down.

- Try to see some humor in the situation: picture the child thrashing about in a three-piece suit, with a briefcase in her hand, for instance.

- Ask another calmer adult to take charge.

Whatever you choose, do not proceed to Level 3 until you really feel you can control your voice, your words, and your actions. "It's always better to do nothing than to overreact to a tantrum or to hurt your child," says Dr. Merritt.

LEVEL 3: IGNORE THE UPROAR

Once you're calm, the next step is to continue what you've already been doing: ignore the tantrum. Don't look at your child, talk to him, or touch him. If he's very young and very out of control, you may want to stand near him, just to reassure him that he's not totally alone with his feelings. If the tantrum seems purely manipulative, however, you should move to another room or another area of the room you're in until the eruption is over. (If you're in a store or other public area, of course, you should never leave your child alone; instead, turn around, or turn your face away.)

Public Tantrums

Public tantrums are the hardest to ignore, but don't let your child figure that out. Even if people you know are looking on with concern or criticism, try to treat a public tantrum exactly as you would a tantrum at home. If you attempt to pacify your child just to avoid a scene, you'll teach her that she can get her way more easily when visitors or strangers are present. There must be no extra benefit to throwing a tantrum in public.

According to most experts, ignoring is the single most effective way to discourage tantrums. The reason is, most of them are thrown for the benefit of an audience. That's why so many kids follow their parents around when they're having a tantrum. Even a 2-year-old can figure out that there's not much point in screaming, yelling, and thrashing about if no one is there to watch and respond.

Tantrum Behavior You CAN Ignore

Breath-holding

You can ignore breath-holding: when a baby or toddler gets so angry he holds his breath until he passes out; his lips may turn blue and his muscles may twitch, though this is not considered seizure activity.

This is the most terrifying of all tantrum behaviors, but it isn't as dangerous as it looks. Even if your child becomes unconscious during a breath-holding spell, he won't die, and it won't damage his brain. Within a minute, his body will relax and he'll automatically start breathing again.

The biggest danger is that you'll be so frightened by seeing your child pass out that you'll rush to his aid and give in to his tantrum. Try to resist this powerful urge, since it only reinforces the behavior. If you can't ignore a breath-holding tantrum:

- Lie your child flat and put a cold, wet washcloth to his forehead (do not shake the child, since that may cause bleeding in the brain)
- As soon as breathing resumes, walk away; tell your child in a matter-of-fact voice that you're sorry you can't help him with this behavior, but that you'll come back as soon as he's recovered
- Even if you are feeling frightened, do not let your child know it
- When the spell is over, give him a brief hug and reassure him that as he grows older, he'll be able to control this behavior himself

• Find something else to do, but do not give in to the tantrum request
• Let your pediatrician know about the breath-holding spells, so she can make sure there are no underlying medical problems or help you with your response strategy.

Call 911 if breathing stops for more than 1 minute and the child does not seem to be regaining consciousness.

Head-banging

You can ignore head-banging: when a child is so angry she bangs her head against the floor, the wall, or some other hard surface.

Head-banging during a tantrum is not a sign of retardation or emotional problems, it does not cause brain damage, and though it looks painful, it is rarely dangerous in any way to normal children. Most kids who do it are smart enough to avoid hurting themselves. They look for surfaces that make lots of noise but cause little pain (such as a hollow wall instead of a concrete floor).

If you fear your child may hurt himself, pick him up and move him to a safer place. But as with other tantrum behaviors, the better you ignore head-banging, the sooner it will go away.

Vomiting

You can ignore vomiting: when a child gets so angry about being ignored during a tantrum that he vomits.

This is not a pretty habit, but it is not dangerous,

either. It does not indicate that you are traumatizing your child by ignoring his tantrum. The best way to respond is to act like the vomiting is no big deal. Clean up the mess in a matter-of-fact way, saying as little as possible, and then continue with your usual tantrum response. Do not let your child feel that he's inconvenienced you or changed your mind in any way.

Unfortunately, as any parent who's tried it knows, it's extremely difficult to ignore a tantrum—especially if it happens in public or with a child whose tantrums are frequent. We have too much vested in wanting our kids to be happy, wanting them to behave, and wanting to feel like good parents to sit by and do nothing. In order to ignore a tantrum, all of those powerful feelings must be set aside; in their place must be a confident belief that by not helping, we're really helping.

This may not feel true—it may even seem cruel to ignore your child when he's in obvious turmoil. But trust me: if you can do it, it works. "Trying to control or stop a tantrum once it's begun is useless," adds Dr. Garber. "It only gives attention to the behavior, and thereby prolongs the outburst." Even a gentle offer to help or make things better is more likely to escalate a tantrum than to dissipate it, he adds. Attention of any kind will encourage future blow-ups.

There's another good reason to ignore tantrums: sometimes, kids (especially younger ones) have no other way to vent their emotions. The tantrum is like an anti-stress safety valve: it allows them to release the pent-up tension and find relief. As long as nothing is being broken and no one is getting hurt, there's no real harm in allowing such an outburst to run its course. As James Windell observes, "You are not an inadequate parent if you allow a tantrum to play itself out."

Tantrum Behavior You CAN'T Ignore

Go directly to Level 4 (hugging, standing by, cooldown time, or time-out) if your child starts:

- Pounding or kicking at things to deliberately damage or break them
- Screaming, yelling, or whining loudly in a quiet public place such as a church, a theater, or a restaurant
- Following you around; scratching, hitting, or kicking you; or clinging to your legs
- Hitting, biting, or hurting another person
- Breaking things
- Throwing objects that could harm others or damage property

Dr. Chess agrees. "I remember once, when my 'difficult' daughter was 3, we were visiting some friends at a summer place," she says. "She wanted something and I said no, so she threw herself on the floor and started kicking and screaming. She was wearing her favorite coat at the time, so I pointed out that the coat was getting dirty. She got up, took the coat off, and then resumed her tantrum. I didn't say another word. I just brushed the coat off and held it until the tantrum was over. Then, when she finished, she retrieved the coat, put it on, and proceeded to have a great day."

If, despite all this, you still think ignoring is too difficult, try the following techniques.

℞ FOR EARLY AND TODDLER TANTRUMS

AGE FLAG: 1 TO 3 YEARS

Distract Your Child

Since very young children tend to lose control over here-and-now issues—they have to leave the park, their cookie just broke, they can't have a toy they want—you can often change their mood just by changing the subject. That doesn't mean giving in to your child, or switching a "no" decision to a "yes"; it means shifting her attention elsewhere so you won't get entangled in a pointless power struggle and her outburst won't overwhelm her. For example, you could:

- Suddenly notice something new or interesting ("Wow, look at how colorful that bird out there is" or "Shh, I hear a funny noise. I wonder what it is.")
- Start doing something fun and invite your child to join in ("I love this book about puppies. I think I'll read it right now. Would you like to read it with me?" or "Mmm, those cookies smell so good I think I'm going to eat one. I wonder if you'd like one too.")
- Arouse her curiosity ("As soon as you're finished crying, we can go outside and see if there's anything new in the garden.")

• Whisper a secret, or start humming your child's favorite song.

Distraction is highly effective with kids this young because they don't carry grudges or wallow in self-pity. Once a tantrum's over, it's over and forgotten; they're happily involved in a new activity. It can also derail a tantrum before it turns too ugly for a parent to easily forget.

℞ FOR PRESCHOOL AND BIG-KID TANTRUMS

AGE FLAG: 3 TO 6 YEARS

Distract Yourself

Older children are more difficult to distract than toddlers. Plus, their language skills are better, so they can use words to engage us more directly in their tantrums ("But you promised me a cookie before dinner"; "That's not fair!"; "You won't let me because you like her better"; "Why can't I have it?").

Resisting the urge to defend ourselves, explain our decisions, or talk our child out of a tantrum is extremely difficult. We tend to think that all we have to do is point out how unreasonable our child is being, and he'll stop the fuss. Children are not as rational as adults, however, and during tantrums they have zero ability to listen and reason. Plus, as Dr. Merritt points out, "Talking, lecturing, and yelling are all forms of attention, and even negative attention fuels tantrums."

For many parents, the best way to resist these incredibly tempting responses is to find something else (anything!) to think about or do. "When our son was about 2," recalls Dr. Garber, "he was a breath-holder. During a tantrum, he'd hold his breath until he passed out. When he came to, he'd check to see if I or my wife was watching, and if we so much as glanced at him, he'd start holding his breath again. We found that the best way to avoid any interaction with him was to act as if we had something else to do—like checking the light fixtures—as soon as a tantrum began."

Other parents have similar strategies. Some, for instance, use tantrum time to:

- Start planning the holiday gift list
- Cut out coupons
- Think about fixing the roof
- Fold or put away the laundry
- Indulge in a happy memory or visualize a beautiful sunset or a favorite friend
- Pick up a book and start to read
- Put on some music

At the very least, you should pretend you're busy, even if all you can think about is what your child is doing and saying. If there's no audience, your tantrum-thrower will eventually get off the stage and find something more interesting to do; as soon as this happens, proceed to Level 5.

If your child's behavior gets worse, however, or you begin to sense that her ability to continue the tantrum exceeds your ability to ignore it, move to Level 4.

Level 4: Contain the Chaos

At Level 4, your only goal is to help your child calm down and regain control, but you need to do this without giving in to the tantrum or letting your child feel that his outburst has had any real effect on you or your decisions. Following are some options.

℞ for Early and Toddler Tantrums

AGE FLAG: 1 TO 3 YEARS

Hugging

Contrary to popular belief, you aren't going to spoil your child by being kind or sympathetic to her when she's throwing a tantrum. While you don't want to hover over her, offer her a bribe, or bend over backward to make the tantrum stop, you can safely offer vital support by quietly hugging, rocking, or snuggling next to her as the outburst unfolds.

"Even if they don't show it, many young children really appreciate being hugged during a tantrum," says Dr. Howard. "If you just walk away from them, they fear that you can't stand their anger and they may feel abandoned—both of which will make the tantrum worse. By hugging, you let the child know that, while you aren't going to give in to her tantrum, you aren't going to desert her either. Children feel more secure just knowing they're near someone who has the ego strength and emotional control they lack."

The only real rule for hugging during a tantrum is to make sure the embrace is loving. (As with "Holding" in Level 1, if you are feeling too angry, this technique will not work.) Also, you'll be more successful if you can stick it out until the tantrum is completely over and the hug becomes mutual. If your child's behavior escalates at first or he resists you, and you respond by throwing up your hands and walking away in disgust, he'll end up feeling even worse.

You shouldn't do a lot of talking while you hug, either, but you may want to repeat a soothing phrase such as "Everything's going to be okay" or "This is so hard" or "I'm going to hold you until you feel better" or "I love you. You'll feel better soon." Be sure not to respond to specific complaints your child has, however, or to engage in any discussions about what caused the tantrum or how your child should be behaving. Your only job at this point is to comfort your child, so she can regain control.

When a Tantrum's in Progress

Words That Work

Try hugging your child and say:

- "You are out of control, and I am going to help you."
- "I'm going to stay right here until you feel better."

Try distracting your child and say:

- "As soon as you are finished crying, we can put on our boots and go play outdoors."
- "Wow, what an interesting-looking bug this is. Come look."

Try ignoring your child and say:

- "I can't decide whether I should vacuum now or just dust."
- "I can't understand you when you're crying, but I'll be happy to listen once you've calmed down."

Call for cool-down time and say:

- "It looks like you need some time alone to calm down."
- "I can see you're feeling really angry. Can you calm yourself down, or do you need to go to your room for a while?"

Words That Don't Work

- "You're too old to have a temper tantrum."
- "Stop that right now."
- "Why are you doing this to me?"
- "You're acting like a spoiled brat."
- "If you don't stop kicking and screaming right this second, you're going to be in *big* trouble."
- "Keep it up and you'll be in time-out for the rest of your life."
- "Please stop crying. Everyone's looking at you, and you're embarrassing me."
- "Here's what you want. Now stop crying."
- "I refuse to stand here and listen to all this noise."

Standing By

If your child is highly resistant to hugging, or you just don't feel you can muster a loving embrace when a tantrum's in progress, simply stand close by and briefly state your support: "I can't talk to you while you're crying, but I'll stay right here until you feel better."

"This won't make the tantrum end, but it will make your child feel significantly safer," says Karen Buchanan.

Dr. Howard agrees. "You shouldn't talk or even look at your child when she's throwing a tantrum," she says, "but you should let her know, by standing nearby, that you aren't going to abandon her in her time of need."

℞ FOR PRESCHOOL AND BIG-KID TANTRUMS

AGE FLAG: 3 TO 6 YEARS

Cool-down Time

By the time your child is 3, he should be learning to calm himself down when a tantrum occurs. A good way to help him practice this skill is to use cool-down time in response to tantrums that just won't end. What this basically entails is sending your child to an unexciting location (the bottom of the stairs, a special chair, the laundry room, or another area of the house) until he's able to act like a human being again. Another alternative, if your child seems too frightened to be alone with his tantrum, is to simply turn away from him while remaining nearby.

Cool-down is not a punishment, and should never be presented as one. It's a way of giving your child the time and space to harness her emotions. As we discussed in Chapters One and Two, most kids can't help themselves when they throw a tantrum—and punishment only makes a melt down worse.

Different experts have different ideas about how to implement cool-down time, but most agree that you must explain the process before you're in a tantrum situation (see "Set Limits" in Chapter Four). In the heat of the moment, you can't expect your child to pick up on a new discipline technique. But if you explain—and even practice—cool-down time beforehand, it will become a logical, predictable response that will actually help your child feel more secure.

In My Experience . . .

The worst way to handle a tantrum . . . "is to shout back at my child. It increases his terror if I lose control just when he needs me to help him get a grip on himself."

What works best for me . . . "is to underplay my reaction, speak in my calmest, most soothing voice, and stay near him—without crowding him. I let him cry himself out for a little bit, but I listen for a slight falter in the intensity of his crying. Then I step in and casually try to distract him. Once his wildness ebbs, then I'll give him a little cuddle and some reassuring talk."

—Holly Hughes
mother of Hugh, age 4,
and Tommy, age 2½

Once you've explained why you'll call cool-down time, and what will happen when you do, follow your plan exactly when a tantrum goes (or threatens to go) into outer orbit. Be sure you include the following steps:

1. Briefly tell your child that cool-down time has begun, and remind him of what he must do (as in: "It's cool-down time. You're having a tantrum, and you need to go to your room, or sit in the cool-down chair, until you're finished crying"). Keep your voice as matter-of-fact as possible and do not say anything else, no matter how hard your child pleads, begs, resists, or complains. Even if he goes for your jugular and says something to the effect of "I hate you. You're the worst mother in the whole world. Everyone hates you," ignore it.

   If he screams "You don't love me" or something similar, you can reassure him briefly, without getting into a debate: "I love you very much, but you are out of control right now, and I'm putting you in cool-down to help you calm down." Otherwise, stay silent.

2. If your child refuses to go into cool-down, calmly pick her up or lead her to the cool-down spot. If she runs away again, repeat the process; do this as often as necessary, until your child complies. (With a younger kid, you can put her in her crib to make sure she stays put; if you're in public, you should take your child to an out-of-the-way bench, a restroom, or the car.)

   If all else fails, put yourself in a cool-down area (inside your room or the bathroom, for instance), and lock the child out (make sure he's safe first). But try to act firm and not angry. Remember, you are not punishing your child, you are giving her space to regain control.

3. Tell your child briefly when cool-down time will be over. This can be anything from "You can come out of cool-down when you've finished crying" to "I'm putting the timer on for 5 minutes, then I'll check to see if your tantrum's over. If it's not, I'll reset the timer for another 5 minutes. If it is over, we can go outside and play." Ignore any attempts at negotiation.

4. If you think it would help to distract him, you could ask your child to count to 10 (or some other number, depending on his abilities), recite a nursery rhyme, sing a song, or take some deep breaths while waiting for cool-down time to end. But make the suggestion briefly and quickly (as in: "Count to 10"; "Sing 'Twinkle, Twinkle' five times"), and don't discuss it at any length.

5. Quickly walk away (to another part of the room or, if your child can handle it, to another room) and find something else to do. If your child knows or suspects that you're still paying attention to his tantrum or listening right outside the door, he'll keep the show going; if he's in another room, he may even kick at the door, throw things around, or make agitating remarks to get you to pop back in and react. Instead, make him think you couldn't care less what he's up to—until he's calm.

6. As soon as your child's been calm for as little as 30 seconds, tell her cool-down time is over—and act like nothing happened. Some kids will want a hug

or kiss to make sure you aren't still holding a grudge, and it's fine to indulge them. But don't lecture, blame, reprimand, call names, yell, accuse, or otherwise discuss your child's infraction. The only requirement for getting out of cool-down time should be ending the tantrum. (You can save any tantrum discussions for later, when you're both feeling less frazzled.) If ending cool-down time releases a new flood of tears, call cool-down again.

7. Within 5 minutes of the tantrum's end, find some reason to praise your child (see Level 5).

If cool-down time doesn't seem to work, it may be because your child needs more help calming down (see "Holding" and Hugging" on pages 134 and 149). Or it may be that your expectations are too high. "Cool-down time and time-out derive much of their power by interrupting an inappropriate behavior, breaking its rhythm, and allowing the parent to redirect what's happening," explains Dr. Williamson. "They are not meant to make your child tremble with fear or to deter misbehavior, but to help him learn his boundaries and improve self-control."

In other words, even if you use cool-down time consistently and correctly, it won't end all tantrums, but it will help you contain those that happen more quickly and more effectively—without igniting a power struggle or damaging anyone's self-esteem.

LEVEL 5: FORGIVE AND FORGET

No matter what the level at which a tantrum ends, do not follow it up with lectures, reprimands, blame, shame, or punishment. A post-tantrum child is already feeling shaken and ashamed of her behavior: you don't have to rub it in. (You can always discuss the outburst later, as part of your prevention strategy; see Chapter Four.)

Instead, as soon as a tantrum ends, shift your attention back to your child and let her know immediately that you still love her. Within 5 minutes, find a reason to praise her for some quality you really value, even if it's a relatively minor one (as in: "I love the way you colored that picture" or "You did a great job setting the table"). You may not be in the mood to think nice things about your child, but you should still force yourself to praise something. By giving more attention to positive behavior than to the tantrum, you motivate your child to seek self-control.

Another good way to follow up a tantrum is to introduce a pleasant activity. Invite your child to share a snack or read a book with you, ask her to help with supper or go for a walk, give her a silent pat on the head when you pass her in the hallway—anything to let her know all's forgiven.

Remember: even if you can't prevent all tantrums, you can make sure that those that happen don't spoil the trust and love you share with your child. In the long run, it's far more important to help your child feel loved and capable than to prove that you're right, to show her who's in charge, or to have a perfectly behaved kid. As Dr. Chess observes: "Behavior problems arise as soon as a child begins seeing his parents as the enemy rather than as people who are on his side and genuinely want him to succeed."

Tantrum Taming at a Glance
Level 1: Is my child safe?

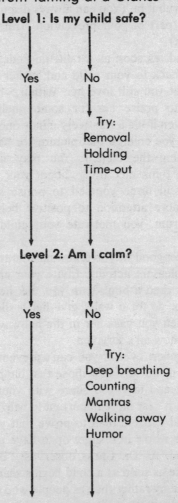

Yes   No

Try:
Removal
Holding
Time-out

Level 2: Am I calm?

Yes   No

Try:
Deep breathing
Counting
Mantras
Walking away
Humor

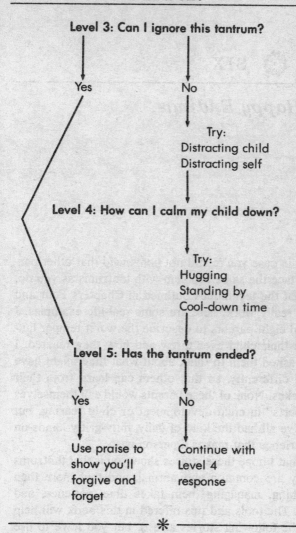

Level 3: Can I ignore this tantrum?

Yes

No

Try:
Distracting child
Distracting self

Level 4: How can I calm my child down?

Try:
Hugging
Standing by
Cool-down time

Level 5: Has the tantrum ended?

Yes

No

Use praise to
show you'll
forgive and
forget

Continue with
Level 4
response

✳

❀ SIX

Happy Endings

Just in case you're still not convinced that other parents face the same problem with tantrums as you do, or that the techniques outlined in Chapters Four and Five really work, here are some real-life examples. I asked eight parents to describe the worst temper tantrum their child ever threw and how they reacted. I also asked them to think about what they might have done differently, so that others can learn from their mistakes. None of these parents would call themselves "experts" in child development or child rearing, but they've all had the kind of daily, nitty-gritty hands-on experience that makes a person wise.

What I hope these stories show you is that tantrums really are common and normal, and that more than anything, managing them takes time, patience, and love. The tools and tips offered in this book will help (as the following stories attest), but you have to use them consistently and conscientiously to make a real impact. This doesn't mean you have to be perfect. If now and then you slip up (parents are, after all, human), your child is unlikely to sustain lasting damage, especially if you can find a way to let him know that no matter what happens, you still love him.

In the end, you are the real expert: the teacher with the most influence on your child's behavior and development. Cherish this job—and use all the resources you can to do it right.

REAL-LIFE TANTRUMS AND HOW THEY ENDED

Early and Toddler Tantrums

AGE FLAG: 1 TO 3 YEARS

THE FOOD MOOD

One recent weekday afternoon, I took my 5-year-old and my 14-month-old to the local library. I had worked during the morning and was feeling rather tired. I knew that both my kids tend to get hungry in inconvenient places at inconvenient times, so I brought plenty of snacks. The first section we visited was the audio-visual department, and while my older son and I were looking for some tapes for him to listen to, my younger son, Tommy, began to get a bit fussy.

I was prepared for this, however: I quickly reached into the diaper bag, pulled out a small box of raisins, opened it up wide so he could feed himself, and handed it to him, certain that I could now return to our search for tapes in peace.

About a minute later, though, Tommy resumed crying, more intensely this time, and I could sense real frustration. When I looked down, I saw that he was having trouble with a bunch of raisins that had gotten clumped together. I took the box from him, so I could open it wider and declump the raisins, and he suddenly started screaming. He arched his back, turned his head away when I tried to give him back the box, then grabbed at the box and threw it onto the floor, shrieking all the while. I offered him a bottle; he became more enraged, squirming from side to side in his stroller.

Finally, I lost my patience; I was angry that nothing I could do seemed to satisfy him in the least, but instead made him even wilder. Our next stop, the children's book section where we usually spend most of our time, seemed impossible with all the embarrassing screaming, and I knew I wouldn't get a chance to get out any books for myself, either. Our afternoon at the library was shot because my son was once again acting like a lunatic.

"That's it," I said bitterly. As fast as I could, I wheeled the stroller outside. Tommy was still screaming, my older son was disappointed, and I was angry. Tommy continued to squirm and twist until he was almost out of the stroller, so I simply unbuckled him and let him stagger around in the courtyard for a while. Eventually, the new environment distracted him, and he calmed down enough to drink some milk. Finally, we were able to return to the library.

In retrospect, I wish I hadn't taken the raisins from him: I might've sensed that he was on the verge of losing it. I also think I should've brought him outside sooner, while I was still fairly calm.

I'm not sure I have any great advice for other parents; both my children have hot tempers, and my own reactions are perhaps not the best model. The advice I'd give applies to myself perhaps most of all: try not to lose your temper when they lose theirs.

—Henry Cunningham
father of William and Tommy

A PUBLIC OUTCRY

One day, when I was pushing my daughter, Mia (then 22 months old) in her stroller, I decided to stop at a David's Cookies store to buy her a treat. I bought some cookies, sat down at a little table, and handed her one. All of a sudden, for some reason, she started screaming. To this day, I'm not sure why—maybe she didn't like the cookie I gave her; maybe I didn't give it to her fast enough. Who knows?

At first, I thought it would help to take her out of the stroller, but as soon as I did, she began acting like a bat out of hell; she seemed to be auditioning for *The Exorcist*. She threw herself down in the middle of the floor and began screaming and kicking. I couldn't even pick her up.

This went on for what seemed like 15 minutes. The people at the other tables couldn't believe their eyes or their ears; I couldn't, either. I thought something was seriously wrong with my daughter. I was so embarrassed, I wanted to die.

Eventually, I was able to lift her up, carry her out, and wrestle her back into her stroller. The whole way home, she continued screaming. Everyone else on the street stared at us. Finally, when we were back in the apartment, she began to calm down. I tried my best to speak to her calmly, and asked if she wanted to watch a video. She nodded, sat down on the couch, and was fine.

I've found that distraction—putting on some kids' music or a video, or even putting a crayon in the child's hand—is really effective in diffusing tantrums. But I also think it's really important for the parent or caregiver to distance herself from what's happening, so you don't react by screaming back. If necessary, pretend that your child belongs to someone else, so you can be more objective about her behavior. If she's just tired or hungry, she probably can't help herself. Give her time to blow off steam, and then, when she's calm, give her extra attention and love.

—Donna Kerbel,
mother of Mia

CALM OR CONSEQUENCES

Zack began throwing tantrums at a very early age, but his worst period was between ages 1½ and 3. Everything was difficult: getting him to come to dinner, getting him to share toys with visiting friends, buying him shoes in a store. We'd have these knock-down, drag-out fights over the most mundane things, and we'd both end up exhausted.

The worst tantrum I remember from that period happened in a clothing store. I had arranged to meet a friend and her children there, and we'd planned to take the kids out for hot dogs at a nearby deli. As the other mother and I greeted each other and began talking, however, Zack became very upset over something (I'm not even sure what it was—maybe one of the other children was doing something he didn't like). Anyway, he began whining, and then he totally lost it. He started kicking and screaming, so I picked him up and took him out to our van, in the hopes that he could collect himself.

He couldn't. He kept on crying and screaming, and then began hitting the windows. In the calmest voice I could muster, I told him that if he couldn't stop hitting the windows and calm down, we would miss lunch with our friends. I gave him a few minutes, but he showed no signs of ending the tantrum, so I followed through and drove him home. I think it was the first time he got a glimmer of the idea that his actions had consequences that weren't always pleasant.

He was still crying as we walked into the house 10 minutes later, so I offered him a snack, and he finally quieted down.

One thing I find really helpful is to have a ritual for making up after a tantrum. Usually, when things are calm, I go to Zack and say, 'Is it time for our make-up kiss?' and he puckers up to kiss me. Then we can start fresh.

I also find it incredibly helpful to talk to other mothers who have tantrum-prone kids—not people who will listen to you and then say, "My kids never have tantrums!", but friends who can reassure you that you're a good, caring mother, and that you're doing the best you can. Tantrums can really shake your confidence: you need that support.

—Carolyn Davenport,
mother of Zack and Ellen

ATTACK OF THE COOKIE MONSTER

One night, just when I was frantically trying to get dinner together, my son, Hugh, then 2½, decided he wanted a cookie. He was hungry and tired to begin with, so when I told him "No cookie, dinner will be ready in 5 minutes," he flung himself at the cabinet where we keep the cookies and began to cry; when I pried him away from there, he threw himself full length on the floor. Then, with great, heaving screams, he scrambled to his feet and launched at me, pummeling me with his fists. He became hysterical. I had to put him in his room and hold the door shut for a while, so he could stop being so angry and want to be with me more than he wanted to hurt me.

At first, I too felt angry and put-upon—until I saw how out of control he was. Then I dropped my self-referential attitude, realized the tantrum had nothing to do with me and had no reflection on my parenting skills, and calmed down instantly. I just felt sorry for him.

I let him out of his room after about a minute and a half and just held him on my lap (he was still kicking and screaming) until he started to run out of steam. Then I said, "Are you ready to get up now? Is it okay if I go fix dinner?" I thought it would help him feel more in control if he were the one to give permission for us to separate. He said yes, and then, sniffling but subdued, went off to play, while I finished cooking.

My advice to other parents dealing with tantrums is don't take them personally. The problem is not you, and it's not a character thing with them. It's a normal part of development. Don't typecast your child, and don't carry a grudge. Instead, try to reconstruct the circumstances that brought on the tantrum, to see if you can circumvent them next time.

Your child will grow out of this phase—unless you let him carve a tantrum groove.

—Holly Hughes,
mother of Hugh and Tommy

Preschool Tantrums

AGE FLAG: 3 TO 4 YEARS

MALL MANIA

My son Sam frequently had tantrums in stores, so I did my best to avoid them when he was with me. But one time, when I couldn't avoid it, he threw the worst tantrum I remember. He was 3 at the time, and it was the day before we were leaving on a trip to visit his grandmother. She had asked me to bring along a toy sprinkler for the kids to play with at her house, so I had to run out to the mall to get one. We managed to find the sprinkler and buy it without any problems— and as I was paying for it, I thought, *Whew, I'm home free*. But then I made the mistake of asking my daughter (who's older than Sam) to carry the sprinkler out of the store. It turns out that Sam wanted to carry it out, but by the time I understood that, it was too late.

No sooner had we left the store when he started screaming and yelling; then he flung himself onto the floor and started kicking, too. He was totally out of control, and, since we were on the first level of the mall, his screams were echoing all the way up to the second floor. People were walking by and staring; some were even peering over the second-floor railing to see what was happening. I wanted to just leave him there.

At first, I tried to get him out of the mall, but I quickly realized he was too out of control. So I sat with his sister on a nearby bench and waited for him to calm down. It took a while. I was quite angry and had to control myself, too. Finally, after about 10 long, loud minutes, Sam exhausted himself. He stood up and walked over to me, and I said, "Are you ready to leave now?" He nodded, and we left.

In retrospect, I don't think I would have done anything differently. It was one of those situations where I couldn't avoid a trip to the store. Sometimes you just have to take a tantrum-prone kid out in public.

My advice to other parents in a similar situation is just do whatever it takes to remain calm yourself. Use mental imaging—pretend you're at the beach or something—to avoid reacting.

Also, in general, make sure you get plenty of exercise and have time to yourself as often as possible. When it comes to tantrums, people often talk about managing the child, but I think it's even more important to learn to manage yourself when they happen. If you're feeling rested and refreshed, you'll react much more reasonably.

—Wendy White-Hensen,
mother of Elizabeth and Sam

NEW-SIBLING STRIKE

My daughter, Margaret, was never much of a problem tantrum-wise, but she did lose it now and then. The worst time was when she was about 3½. By then, her younger sister, Charlotte, was a year old and becoming more of a threat. This particular morning, we were in the car, on our way to the library. I decided to dole out some snacks, but I had only brought one banana for both girls to share.

Margaret suddenly began screaming that she wanted her own banana. Of course, I think the real issue was anger over having to share so many things (food, toys, parental attention) with a sibling. She had had enough of this, so she screamed and kicked the back of the seat all the way to the library. When we reached the library, she screamed some more, and kicked at the wall of the building.

It would clearly not have been a good idea to go in, so I carried her kicking and screaming back to the car. It took me 10 minutes to get her secured in her carseat. She continued to scream, and wriggled out of her carseat six times during the (normally) 15-minute ride home. I kept having to pull over and force her back into her carseat.

I was furious that she was acting so completely irrational and that she had spoiled our outing. I reacted tensely, but somehow managed to keep my voice calm as I repeated the same phrase over and over: "I know you are angry, but you still have to stay in your carseat."

When we finally arrived home, I made her a huge lunch with scrambled eggs and cheese, toast, milk, and fruit. (I suspected that one of the reasons for the tantrum might have been that she had eaten pancakes for breakfast, and her blood sugar was low.) After she had eaten her lunch, I put her down for a nap and she slept for hours.

In retrospect, the only thing I wish I'd done differently was turn the car around the minute she started acting up.

In general, though, what helps me most when my kids have tantrums is remembering that they are not an indication of a horrible character flaw, but part of a normal stage of development. I try to focus on the fact that the child is growing and changing, and that tantrums indicate a healthy desire for greater autonomy. I often think things like *Yes, this feisty, independent 3-year-old is sometimes hard to take, but won't she be a terrific 30-year-old!*

—Elizabeth Dunn,
mother of Margaret and Charlotte

AN UNEXPECTED OUTBURST

My first child never threw tantrums—that just wasn't his style. So when my second child came along and did throw them, it was unnerving. I wasn't sure why they were happening (was I giving her too little attention?) or, very often, what to do.

The problem wasn't that Kathy had a lot of tantrums, but the ones she had were very dramatic and unpredictable. I remember one time, when she was 3, she, her sister, her brother, and I were in a store doing some Christmas shopping. She had to go to the bathroom, so I took her to the restroom, but the public toilet was filthy. I told her I needed to clean it off or put paper on the seat before she sat down, and she went off. She started screaming and crying out of utter frustration (though I'm still not sure what she was frustrated about!).

I couldn't get her to calm down, so I finally just picked her up, put her under my arm, and walked out of the store. She was kicking and thrashing, and screaming—in this terrible, shrill voice—things like "Put me down. I hate you." I knew she didn't mean it; she was just out of control.

I, of course, was embarrassed; all I wanted to do was get home. I was angry, too, because I wasn't sure how or why things had fallen apart. It wasn't a "tired" part of the day for her, she wasn't hungry, and I wasn't saying no to something she wanted.

All the way home, she was screaming at the top of her lungs. I had a hard time driving, and at one point, I lost my temper and yelled "Be quiet!" But that was ridiculous—by that time, she was too out of control to quiet down.

When we got home, I took her out of the car, carried her up to her room, and put her on her bed. I wanted to put some distance between the two of us. She cried and cried until she was finally able to calm down.

Then, I hugged her for a long time. Afterward, she went to the bathroom, and we found something else to do.

For me, staying calm is the most important thing when there's a tantrum in progress. I try to remember that the tantrum is more uncomfortable for my child than it is for me, and I remind myself that tantrums don't last forever. I know that if I can stay calm, my child won't get as upset.

> —Kelly Smith,
> mother of James, Kathy, and Lillith

Big-Kid Tantrums

AGE FLAG: 4 YEARS AND UP

A PAINFUL PARTING

When my son Ross was about 4½, he went through a stage where he was throwing two or three tantrums a week. One day, when he was playing outside in the front yard with a friend, he became very abruptly upset because his playmate's mother pulled up in the car to take her son home. He wanted his friend to stay and continue to play.

First he started crying and begging the woman not to take his friend home yet. Then he progressed to screaming, and even tried to run into the street as his friend rode away. As I picked him up and took him into the garage, he became very physical—kicking and resisting me. I restrained him until our garage door closed, then released him. He remained in the garage, kicking the door and screaming. This went on for about 10 minutes—though, at the time, it felt like 4 hours!

I was surprised at the severity of the tantrum, and a little perplexed as to what to do about it. I watched him as he was in the garage (from the kitchen), to make sure he didn't hurt himself, and just waited for him to be finished with it.

When he had completely exhausted himself, he came to me on his own. As usual for him, he was very cuddly and loving after the tantrum, and sat on my lap for several minutes, resting and snuggling. This often happens after he's had a tantrum—it's like I get to see the worst of him for a while, and then, suddenly, the best. After we snuggled for a few moments, he was able to verbalize his frustration and talk with me logically about why he was upset.

I think that if I had given Ross advance warning that his friend's mother was about to arrive ("Ben's mom will be here in about 5 minutes to pick him up"), it would have helped. He tends to adjust to transitions and shift gears more easily when I let him know exactly what's going to happen before it happens. It also helps to give him lots of choices ("Would you rather pick up your toys now, or after supper?"), so he can feel a greater sense of control in his life.

—Trudy Eaton,
mother of Sara and Ross

A HAPPIER BIRTHDAY

Once again, it was supposed to be a happy day. My son Gus was turning 5—and I was determined not to have a repeat of his fourth birthday (the scene I described at the beginning of this book). Weeks before his party—another wonderful event, this time with a clown—I began preparing him for what would happen: who was invited, what we would do, what the clown would be like, and so on. We also talked about how he had lost control the previous year, and together came up with a plan: we'd decorate a special box for the gifts, and he wouldn't open any of them until after the party ended.

Gus was ready—and so was I. But then I got too confident: I allowed Gus to invite his very best friend Aaron to sleep over our house the night before the party. They went to bed at a surprisingly decent hour, but awoke full of excitement at the very crack of dawn. By the time the party started, at 10 A.M., both boys were exhausted.

At one point, in the middle of a rollicking game of tag, Aaron hit Gus on the back, and Gus whipped around and started yelling at him. The two of them were right on the edge of losing it—not because they were really mad at each other, but because they both were tired and the excitement of the party was getting to them.

Once again, as happened the previous year, everything stopped and all eyes turned toward me and Gus. But this time, I wasn't embarrassed: I was prepared. In a calm, matter-of-fact voice, I said, "I think we need a break." Then I led the two tearful boys over to the steps and told them to take some deep breaths. To make sure the breaths were deep and relaxing, I asked them to try and blow my friend, Daniel (who was standing in front of them), clear off the steps. Daniel, of course, hammed up his reaction by first wavering, then tipping, and finally, with perfect sound effects, tumbling off the steps. Within minutes, the boys were laughing and feeling miraculously refreshed.

There was no more arguing that day—and not one tiny little tantrum. Once the other guests had left, Gus tore into his presents, and he and Aaron played blissfully for the rest of the afternoon. I felt relieved and proud. My son had reached a milestone—a tantrum-free birthday—and (thanks to all the experts and parents I interviewed for this book) I had been able to help.

There's only one more thing I can tell you I know is absolutely true about tantrums, based on my own experience: the tantrum years do end, and no matter how bad things get, you and your child can survive them. Three years ago, I would never have believed that my temperamental 2-year-old would grow into a sensitive, caring, self-controlled kid. But at age 5, Gus is all that and more. He can still lose his temper—especially when he's sick or tired out from a full day of play—but nowadays it's rare, and we both know how to react so that things don't turn ugly.

I wish I could add that tantrums are a thing of the past in my household, but I can't: Teddy's almost 2 and is already showing signs of being more temperamental than his big brother.

This time, at least, I'll know what to do!

Resources

BOOKS

Brazelton, T. Berry, M.D. *Touchpoints*. Addison-Wesley, 1994

Chess, Stella, M.D., and Thomas, Alexander, M.D. *Know Your Child*. Basic Books, 1987

Galinsky, Ellen, and David, Judy. *The Preschool Years*. Ballantine Books, 1991

Garber, Stephen W., Ph.D., Garber, Marianne Daniels, Ph.D., and Spizman, Robyn Freedman. *Monsters Under the Bed and Other Childhood Fears*. New York: Villard Books, 1993, and *Good Behavior*. New York: St. Martin's Paperbacks, 1991

Green, Christopher, M.D. *Toddler Taming*. Ballantine Books, 1985

Kelly, Jeffrey, M.D. *Solving Your Child's Behavior Problems, an Everyday Guide for Parents*. Little, Brown, 1983

Pantell, Robert H., M.D., Fries, James F., M.D., and Vickery, Donald M., M.D. *Taking Care of Your Child.* Addison-Wesley, 1990

Rothbart, Mary K., and Mauro, Jennifer Alansky. "Questionnaire Approaches to the Study of Infant Temperament," *Individual Differences in Infancy: Reliability, Stability, Prediction.* Erlbaum, 1990

Samalin, Nancy, and Whitney, Catharine. *Love and Anger: The Parental Dilemma.* Viking Penguin, 1991

Schmitt, Barton D., M.D., FAAP. *Your Child's Health.* Bantam, 1991

Shelov, Steven P., M.D. (editor). *Caring for Your Baby and Young Child: Birth to Age 5.* Bantam, 1991

Spock, Benjamin, M.D., and Rothenberg, Michael B., M.D. *Dr. Spock's Baby and Child Care.* Pocket Books, 1985

Turecki, Stanley, M.D., and Tonner, Leslie. *The Difficult Child.* Bantam, 1989

Williamson, Peter, Ph.D. *Good Kids, Bad Behavior.* Simon & Schuster, 1991

Windell, James. *8 Weeks to a Well-Behaved Child.* Macmillan, 1994, and *Discipline: A Sourcebook of 50 Failsafe Techniques for Parents.* Collier Books, 1991

ARTICLES

Arbetter, Sandra R., MSW. "The Many Faces of Anger," *Current Health* 2, January 1990

Eberlein, Tamara. "Can You Discipline a Baby?" *American Baby,* September 1993; "Cooling Off a Hotheaded Kid," *Redbook,* November 1991; and "Do You Have a Difficult Child?" *American Baby,* May 1992

Gibson, Janice T., Ed.D. "Coping with a Difficult Child," *Parents,* November 1987

Israeloff, Roberta. "Meltdown," *Parents,* August 1994

LaForge, Ann E. "Punishments That Fit the Crime," *Child,* November 1994, and "6 Temper Tantrum Tactics," *Child,* June/July 1992

Lally, J. Ronald, Ed.D. "Don't Label Your Child," *Parents,* October 1993

Marks, Jane. "Abby's Story," *Parents,* April 1991, and "Angry Alan, Sulky Sue & Cranky Craig," *Parents,* October 1986

Morse, Michele Block. "Fitting into the Family," *Parents,* July 1990

Rosenberg, Janice. "Are You and Your Baby An Odd Couple?" *American Baby,* November 1992

Rubenstein, Carin, Ph.D. "Mad as H--L," *Child,* April 1992

Schmitt, Barton D., M.D., FAAP. "Big-Kid Tantrums," *Child,* December/January 1994

Segal, Julius. "I'm So Angry!" *Parents,* August 1988

Siegler, Ava L., Ph.D. "Short-Fuse Kids," *Child,* February 1994, and "Are You Being Manipulated?" *Child,* November 1992

Spock, Benjamin, M.D. "Good Ways to Handle a Child's Anger," *Redbook,* December 1989

Waters, Marjorie. "Sensitive Kids," *Parents,* November 1990

Weissbourd, Bernice. "Coping with Tantrums and Tears," *Parents,* February 1992, and "Temper Tantrums," *Parents,* October 1989

For a free copy of the brochure "Temper Tantrums: A Normal Part of Growing Up," send a self-addressed, stamped envelope to the American Academy of Pediatrics, Dept. C, 141 Northwest Point Blvd., P.O. Box 927, Elk Grove Village, IL 60009-0927.

About the Author

Ann E. LaForge is a contributing editor at *Child* magazine. She has written hundreds of articles on children, health, parenting, psychology, and other topics for numerous national publications, including *The New York Times*, *Redbook*, *Good Housekeeping*, *Healthy Kids*, *Glamour*, *Bride's*, and *Bridal Guide*. She has also won awards for her coverage of family issues within the field of business motivation.

Ann lives in Durham, North Carolina, with her husband, and two wild but wonderful sons, who have helped her become an expert on temper tantrums.